Joint Commission

S *BHC*

1999–2000 Standards for Behavioral Health Care

- Accreditation Policies
- Standards
- Intents

Joint Commission Mission

The mission of the Joint Commission on Accreditation of Healthcare Organizations is to improve the quality of care provided to the public through the provision of health care accreditation and related services that support performance improvement in health care organizations.

Joint Commission educational programs and publications support, but are separate from, the accreditation activities of the Joint Commission. Attendees at Joint Commission educational programs and purchasers of Joint Commission publications receive no special consideration or treatment in, or confidential information about, the accreditation process.

Printed in the U.S.A.

Requests for permission to make copies of any part of this work should be mailed to:
Permissions Editor
Department of Publications
Joint Commission on Accreditation of Healthcare Organizations
One Renaissance Boulevard
Oakbrook Terrace, Illinois 60181

ISBN: 0-86688-594-3
Library of Congress Catalog Number: 98-89671

For more information about the Joint Commission, please contact our Web site at
http://www.jcaho.org

Contents

Introduction

The *1999–2000 Standards for Behavioral Health Care* includes standards, intent statements, and accreditation policies and procedures. The standards-related information is provided in an integrated format to help you better understand the expectations of each standard in the accreditation process. Additional chapters explain how to use the standards-related information, including how to use standards and indicators together to measure and improve performance.

This introduction is designed to provide you with information on the following topics:

- New materials for this edition, including chapters, features, and standards;
- Surveyor laptop technology and the survey process; and
- Accreditation process initiatives: continuous accreditation and the use of performance measures in the accreditation process.

For the purpose of readability and ease of use, this introduction is organized in a question-and-answer format.

What's New in the *SBHC*?

Changes to the *SBHC* are made in response to suggestions from customers and relate to important issues that clearly support quality individual care. In the past year, many chapters have been revised and improved to include additional information requested by customers. Table 1, page 2, summarizes the major revisions that occurred for this 1999–2000 edition.

How Is New Technology Enhancing the Accreditation Survey Process?

The Surveyor Laptop Technology Project

In summer 1998, the Joint Commission implemented surveyor laptop technology into the survey process. Surveyors now use laptop computers to enter their survey findings on site. The laptop computers are equipped with specially designed decision-support software. The software is designed to

- improve the validity and reliability of the survey results;
- enable surveyors to provide behavioral health care organizations with a preliminary report on site at the end of the survey; and
- reduce turnaround time on the behavioral health care organization's final accreditation report.

Each surveyor gathers and inputs data into the laptop computer. The special software guides the gathering of data, integrates surveyors' findings, scores the standards, aggregates scores, and compiles a draft survey report. Since the software completes the scoring, the reliability and validity of the accreditation process are significantly improved.

Preliminary Reports. Among the advantages of the surveyor laptop technology is the production of a draft accreditation decision report for review before the surveyor leaves the behavioral health care organization. This preliminary report is provided to the behavioral health care organization's chief executive officer and used during the surveyor's presentation of the survey findings at the Leadership Exit Conference. These reports are preliminary; the final *Official Accreditation Decision Report* may differ from the preliminary report. A final accreditation decision is made following review of the survey findings at the Joint Commission's central office. This process is designed to minimize and, in most cases, eliminate the differences between the preliminary and final reports.

The Joint Commission cautions behavioral health care organizations that want to make their preliminary reports public that the preliminary report is *not* a final decision. Behavioral health care organizations

Table 1. Summary of Major Revisions to the *CAMBHC* for 1999–2000

Chapter	Content Summary
Introduction	Provides you with new information for this edition, including chapters, features, and standards, surveyor laptop technology and the survey process, and accreditation process initiatives, such as the use of performance measures in the accreditation process
The Accreditation Cycle	Formerly "Accreditation Policies and Procedures." Revised chapter addresses revised Sentinel Event Policy and other compliance issues; includes sample application
Accreditation Participation Requirements	New chapter addressing ongoing requirements for continued participation in the accreditation process
Rights, Responsibilities, and Ethics (RI)	Added a new standard (RI.8.4) addressing the integrity of clinical decision making
Assessment (PE)	Minor standards and intent statement revisions for clarity
Care (TX)	Revised and renumbered standards for ease in understanding and implementing standards New standards on administering medication Revised intent statements for clarity
Improving Organization Performance (PI)	Revised standards to emphasize: ■ Data analysis as opposed to data assessment ■ Analysis of sentinel events and reducing risk thereof ■ Sustained improvement New definition of perception of care (formerly "satisfaction")
Leadership (LD)	Revised intent statements for clarity
Management of the Environment of Care (EC)	Revised standard on information collection and evaluation Revised intent statements for clarity
Management of Human Resources (HR)	Revised standards Revised intent statements for clarity
Management of Information (IM)	Restructuring of standards regarding verbal orders

continued on next page

Table 1. Summary of Major Revisions to the *CAMBHC* for 1999–2000 (continued)

Chapter	Content Summary
Surveillance, Prevention, and Control of Infection (IC)	Revised overview Revised and renumbered standards Revised intent statements for clarity
Behavioral Health Promotion (PS)	New chapter emphasizing behavioral health promotion with three new standards for those organizations who consider behavioral health promotion as part of their mission.
Glossary	Revised to incorporate more contemporary definitions of terms used throughout the manual

are encouraged to use the preliminary report for quality improvement purposes only. However, if a behavioral health care organization chooses to publicize its preliminary report, it should emphasize that the findings are preliminary.

The Joint Commission will not comment to members of the news media or community on the findings and decision reflected in the preliminary report. The accreditation decision and report are official only after the final accreditation decision report is sent to the organization.

Web Site. The Joint Commission's award-winning Web site (http://www.jcaho.org) is a valuable resource for organizations. It provides

- up-to-date information about Joint Commission initiatives, including ORYX;
- a complete collection of ORYX listed performance measurement systems with links to their Web sites and a list of candidate systems for ORYX;
- information about accreditation programs;
- an electronic version of the *National Library of Healthcare Indicators,* a collection of 225 performance measure indicators judged to have face-validity; and
- other news and information.

A complete directory of Joint Commission accredited organizations is also available on the Web site. This new directory, Quality Check™, includes the following information for each accredited health care organization:

- Organization name, address, telephone number, and Web site address with e-mail contact, if available;
- Accreditation decision based on the most recent full survey and accreditation date;
- Current accreditation status and accreditation status effective date; and
- An easy-to-use, printable performance report (1996, 1997, and future reports).

The Joint Commission's Web site address is http://www.jcaho.org.

What is Continuous Accreditation? Why Should My Behavioral Health Care Organization Be Interested in It?

Continuous accreditation refers to the process by which an organization continuously evaluates and improves its processes to maintain performance that constantly meets or exceeds accreditation requirements. The Joint Commission is committed to helping organizations move toward continuous accreditation.

For some behavioral health care organizations accredited by the Joint Commission, the accreditation process involves a three-year performance measurement and improvement cycle driven by the timing of the triennial survey. In the 12 months prior to the survey, an organization may devote considerable resources to getting ready for the survey. Performance improvement efforts may be undertaken and results measured in order to meet survey requirements. Upon completion of the survey, the organization may return to "business as usual" and may reduce its focus on performance improvement efforts.

By participating in continuous accreditation efforts, organizations monitor and improve their performance on a year-round, year-in-and-year-out basis. At any point in their triennial accreditation cycle, organizations know how they are doing, are aware of its performance areas, and know whether performance improvement efforts are achieving the desired results. Continuous improvement efforts help organizations maintain the highest possible quality of patient care and services. In addition, organizations can use their resources more wisely, avoiding the high cost of "gearing up" for a Joint Commission survey.

Behavioral health care organizations interested in continuous accreditation efforts can perform continuous self-assessment using the accreditation standards in this manual. The *SBHC* provides a tool for ongoing self-evaluation against nationally recognized standards. Behavioral health care organizations may wish to focus on one or two chapters each month to review their processes and evaluate their progress with performance improvement initiatives. This kind of continuous self-assessment helps organizations prepare for their Joint Commission survey by maintaining readiness on an ongoing basis.

How Will the Use of Performance Measures Be Integrated in the Accreditation Process?

The Joint Commission's current triennial, on-site survey process is evolving to include performance measurement data to continually assure the public and other interested stakeholders that continuous attention is being given to the care provided by health care organizations.

Following the data submission to the Joint Commission, Joint Commission staff will use criteria to review data trends and determine if contact with the health care organization is indicated (for example, a phone call, a request for a written progress report, or an on-site survey). Such reviews will begin once enough data points are available, presumably by the end of 2000. Particular attention will be given to the way in which the health care organization uses the data to analyze processes and improve care. In addition, a summary of organization performance data will be provided to surveyors for use during the regular on-site triennial survey.

The Accreditation Cycle: Official Accreditation Policies and Procedures

Chapter Overview

This chapter provides information relevant to all behavioral health care organizations interested in Joint Commission accreditation, whether they are applying for the first time or on a renewal basis. The chapter describes the Joint Commission's official accreditation policies and procedures. They apply to all organizations either currently accredited by, or seeking accreditation by, the Joint Commission.

The chapter includes information relevant to behavioral health care organizations

- *at all times* (general information), including accreditation eligibility; survey scope, options, and fees; and information, and public information policies;
- *before the survey,* including an overview of the survey process, survey application and scheduling, the survey team and agenda, notifying the public about a Joint Commission survey, and conducting public information interviews;
- *during the survey,* including how the Joint Commission handles individual care or safety concerns, on-site survey activities, the use of laptop technology during the survey, and preliminary accreditation reports;
- *following the survey,* including accreditation decisions, survey report revision requests, and decision appeals; and
- *before the next survey,* including monitoring between surveys, the duration of accreditation awards, the accreditation renewal process, notification of organization changes between surveys, and unscheduled and unannounced surveys.

The chapter is organized into major sections reflecting these categories. You will be able to locate the policies and procedures applicable to your organization according to where your organization is in the accreditation process or cycle. An organization must follow the policies and procedures described in this chapter in order to participate and continue to participate in the accreditation process. An organization that fails to follow the policies and procedures described in this chapter may be considered to have withdrawn from the accreditation process.

Note: *The "Accreditation Participation Requirements" chapter (pages 39 through 44) includes specific requirements for accreditation participation. Requirements 1 through 3 and 7 through 10 are existing policies within this "Accreditation Cycle" chapter and are currently effective for accreditation purposes. Cross-references to the accreditation participation requirements can be found in the applicable sections of this chapter.*

General Information

This section provides information relevant to an organization either applying for Joint Commission accreditation or seeking continued accreditation. Since this material is revised on a regular basis, all organizations are encouraged to review it.

Organizations Eligible for Survey

General Eligibility Requirements. Any organization may apply for a Joint Commission accreditation survey under the standards in this manual* if the following requirements are met:

- The organization is in the United States or its territories or, if outside the United States, is operated by the United States government, under a charter of the United States Congress, or for other organizations outside of the United States that meet the following criteria:
  - The nature of the health care practices in the applicant organization is compatible with the intents of Joint Commission standards;
  - With the use of available translators, as necessary, the surveyors can effectively communicate with substantially all of the organization's management and clinical personnel and at least half of the organization's individuals, and can understand medical records and documents that relate to the organization's performance; or
  - United States citizens make up at least 10% of the organization's individual population

    OR

    A United States government agency contracts with the organization to provide services to United States citizens

    OR

    United States citizens preferentially use the organization in that country.
- The organization assesses and improves the quality of its services. This process includes a review of care by clinicians, when appropriate.
- The organization identifies the services it provides, indicating which services it provides directly, under contract, or through some other arrangement.
- The organization provides services addressed by the Joint Commission's standards.

Purpose of a Survey

A Joint Commission accreditation survey provides an assessment of an organization's compliance with standards and their intent statements developed by the Joint Commission. The Joint Commission evaluates an organization's compliance based on

- verbal information provided to the Joint Commission;
- on-site observations by Joint Commission surveyors; and
- documents provided by the organization.

The survey is key to accreditation. The Joint Commission's accreditation process seeks to help organizations identify and correct problems and improve the quality of care and services provided. In addition to evaluating compliance with standards and their intent statements, significant time is spent in consultation and education.

Scope of Accreditation Surveys

General Survey Categories. The Joint Commission surveys and accredits health care organizations using standards from one or more of the following manuals:

- *Accreditation Manual for Preferred Provider Organizations*;
- *Comprehensive Accreditation Manual for Ambulatory Care*;
- *Comprehensive Accreditation Manual for Behavioral Health Care*;
- *Comprehensive Accreditation Manual for Health Care Networks*;
- *Comprehensive Accreditation Manual for Home Care*;
- *Comprehensive Accreditation Manual for Hospitals: The Official Handbook*;

* The Joint Commission will work with the organization to determine which standards from other accreditation programs are applicable.

- *Comprehensive Accreditation Manual for Long Term Care* (includes standards for dementia special care units and subacute care programs);
- *Comprehensive Accreditation Manual for Long Term Care Pharmacies*;
- *Comprehensive Accreditation Manual for Managed Behavioral Health Care*; and
- *Comprehensive Accreditation Manual for Pathology and Clinical Laboratory Services.*

Tailored Surveys. The Joint Commission tailors its survey to reflect the services offered by the organization. The Joint Commission creates a tailored survey for an organization providing services covered by standards in more than one of the accreditation manuals listed above. The tailored survey will be based on the services provided by the organization as reported in its Application for Survey. The Joint Commission provides the organization with a copy of each of the manuals to be used in the survey before it is conducted. The Joint Commission determines which manuals are applicable based on information provided in the Application for Survey.

Integrated Survey Process. In January 1998, the Joint Commission launched the Integrated Survey Process (ISP) for small hospitals with an average daily census of less than 40 that have long term care and/or home care services. The ISP reduces duplication by offering a single survey with a single team of surveyors and replaces the tailored survey process, which requires additional surveyors for additional components evaluated in small hospitals. The new process includes evaluating performance in those functions that are common across the hospital's components once for the entire organization. Through the ISP, small hospitals with one additional component (long term care or home care services) will be surveyed by two surveyors for three days. Small hospitals with both of these components will be surveyed by two surveyors for four days. Beginning in January 1999, the ISP will be extended to include behavioral health care components (partial hospitalization and residential services) in small hospitals and all psychiatric hospitals regardless of size. The ISP will be expanded to include additional settings in the future.

Single Accreditation Awards. The Joint Commission survey, assuming satisfactory compliance, provides one accreditation award for all of the organization's services, programs, and related organizations. Included in each organization's survey and accreditation decision are all services, programs, and related organizations that are

- organizationally and functionally integrated or
- publicly represented as a part of the organization.

Organizational and functional integration refer to the degree to which the service, program, or related entity is owned and operated by the applicant organization. A service, program, or related entity is any organized health care delivery site that is eligible for survey. For example, these include satellite clinics operated away from the main organization site.

Organizational integration exists when the applicant organization's governing body, either directly or ultimately, controls budgetary and resource allocation decisions for both the applicant organization *and* the service, program, or related entity included in the survey. Organizational integration also exists when separate corporate entities share more than 50% of the same governing body membership.

Functional integration exists when the entity meets three of the following criteria, including criterion 1 or 2:

1. The applicant organization and the service, program, or related entity
   - use the same process for determining membership of licensed independent practitioners in practitioner panels or medical or professional staff or
   - have a common organized medical or professional staff.
2. The applicant organization's human resources function hires and assigns staff at the service, program, or related entity and has the authority to

- terminate staff at the entity,
- transfer staff between the applicant organization and the entity, and
- conduct performance appraisals of the staff who work in the entity.

3. With few exceptions, the applicant organization's policies and procedures are applicable to the service, program, or related entity.
4. The applicant organization manages significant operations of the service, program, or related entity; that is, the service, program, or related entity has little or no management authority or autonomy independent of the applicant organization.
5. The service, program, or related entity's individual records are integrated in the applicant organization's individual record system.
6. The applicant organization applies its performance improvement program to the entity and has authority to implement actions intended to improve performance at the service, program, or related entity.
7. The applicant organization bills for services provided by the service, program, or related entity under the name of the applicant organization.

The Joint Commission assesses an organization's public representation of its services by examining letterhead, brochures, telephone book listings, and other advertising media. Commonality of names may also be relevant.

The Joint Commission evaluates all health care services provided by the organization for which the Joint Commission has standards and makes one accreditation decision and survey report. An organization must be prepared to provide evidence of its compliance with each applicable standard. To gain accreditation, an organization must demonstrate *overall* compliance with the standards and their intent statements, not necessarily compliance with *each* standard and its intent statement.

Contracted Services. The Joint Commission evaluates the organization's assessment of the quality of services provided under contractual arrangements. The Joint Commission reserves the right to evaluate, as part of its survey, services provided by another organization or provider. However, the Joint Commission will not ordinarily do so if the contracted organization is separately accredited by the Joint Commission. It may, however, survey performance issues between the contracted organization and the applicant organization, regardless of the accreditation status of the contracted organization. The Joint Commission also surveys services provided on site under contract.

Multiorganization Option

The Joint Commission offers multiorganization* systems that own or operate at least two organizations the option of a modified survey process. This option has three components:

- A corporate orientation;
- A consecutive survey of participating organizations with the same survey team leader; and
- A corporate summation.

A system may choose to have either a corporate orientation, a corporate summation, or both. The orientation session provides an opportunity for corporate staff to orient the survey team to the structure and practices of the system. The survey team will also survey centralized corporate services, documentation, and policies and procedures applicable to Joint Commission standards. The corporate summation provides an overall analysis of the system's strengths and weaknesses. It also

* **multiorganization survey option** A survey option of the Joint Commission that is available to a single corporation or governmental agency that operates or governs two or more health care organizations. The survey includes a corporate orientation; a consecutive survey of participating organizations with the same team leader; a separate survey, accreditation decision, and certificate for each member organization; and a corporate summation conference.

provides consultation and education related to accreditation survey findings across the system. There is a separate fee for the corporate orientation and corporate summation.

Continuity in the composition of the survey team will be maintained by the survey team leader. The remaining members of the survey team will rotate every third or fourth survey, depending on the location of the organizations being surveyed. The survey team leader will compile the information necessary to support the corporate summation.

A rotating surveyor is selected to survey an organization within a system based on the region in which the organization is located and to which the surveyor is assigned. Therefore, although the team leader may cross geographic regions and survey outside of his or her assigned region, rotating surveyors will be selected to survey system organizations only within their assigned region.

Through the multiorganization option, the Joint Commission accredits the individual health care organizations that are part of a multiorganization system, not the system itself. Therefore, each organization within a system will receive its own accreditation decision and report. The findings and decision for one organization within a system will have no bearing on those of another organization within the system.

Early Survey Policy

An organization wishing to be accredited by the Joint Commission may choose one of two Early Survey Policy Options described here. Under both Option 1 and Option 2, organizations are required to undergo two surveys. However, the nature of the surveys and the potential outcomes differ. The first survey under Option 2 is a full accreditation survey, rather than the more limited first survey under Option 1.

The Public Information Policy (pages 19 through 22) applies to both Option 1 and Option 2 described above.

The sidebar (page 11) highlights Early Survey Options 1 and 2 and describes the potential outcomes of each survey.

Option 1 (Provisional Accreditation)

A. *Eligibility.* This option is available to any organization that is currently not accredited *except* an organization that has been denied accreditation because it provided falsified information within the past year. Organizations must declare during the application process that they wish to be surveyed under this option.

B. *The First Survey.* When an organization chooses Option 1, the Joint Commission will conduct two on-site surveys. It can conduct the first survey as early as two months before the organization begins operating, provided it meets the following criteria:
   - It is licensed or has a provisional license, according to applicable law and regulation;
   - The building in which the services will be offered or from which the services will be coordinated is identified, constructed, and equipped to support such services;
   - It has identified its chief executive officer (CEO) or administrator and its clinical director; and
   - It has identified the date it will begin operations.

   Generally, the first survey uses a limited set of standards and assesses only the organization's physical facilities, policies and procedures, plans, and related structural considerations.

C. *Provisional Accreditation.* The Joint Commission grants provisional accreditation to an organization in overall compliance with the standards and their intent statements assessed in the first survey under Early Survey Option 1. An organization *not* in overall compliance must reapply and begin the accreditation process again. An organization that meets the decision rules for conditional accreditation will also be granted provisional accreditation status.

The provisional accreditation decision will include assignment of a "special type I recommendation" indicating the requirement for survey against the full set of applicable standards, including all track record requirements. Other type I recommendations may also be assigned based on survey findings from the first survey.

For an organization operating when the survey is conducted, the effective date for its provisional accreditation status is the day after the survey was conducted. For an organization not in operation, the effective date is the day after it begins operating. If the organization is not in operation at the time of survey, the organization must confirm in writing the date it begins operating.

Provisional accreditation status remains until the organization has completed a second, full survey or the Joint Commission has withdrawn the provisional accreditation. The Joint Commission may withdraw provisional accreditation

- when an organization that was not providing services at the time of the first survey does not begin services when expected;
- if an organization does not meet the survey eligibility criteria (see page 6); or
- if an organization fails to accept the date of the second survey.

In these cases, the organization must begin the accreditation process again.

D. *The Second Survey.* The second survey is a full accreditation survey. The Joint Commission conducts this survey

- approximately six months after the first survey; and
- at least four months after the organization has begun operating.

The organization's accreditation status, based on survey results, will change to

- accreditation with commendation;
- accreditation;
- accreditation with type I recommendations;
- conditional accreditation;
- preliminary nonaccreditation; or
- not accredited.

The effective date of the accreditation decision is the day after the *second* survey.

A type I recommendation(s) addresses insufficient or unsatisfactory compliance with standards and their intent statements in a specific performance area. An organization receiving any such recommendations is required to resolve them within specified time frames to remain accredited. The organization's three-year accreditation cycle begins the day after the second survey was conducted, unless the Joint Commission reached a decision not to accredit.

Option 2

A. *Eligibility.* Option 2 is available only to an organization that has

- never been surveyed by the Joint Commission;
- been in actual operation for at least one month; and
- cared for at least ten individuals by the time of the first survey with at least one individual in active treatment at the time of survey.

B. *The First Survey.* When an organization chooses Option 2, the Joint Commission will conduct an initial full accreditation survey. If the organization demonstrates satisfactory compliance with standards and their intent statements in the first survey, it will be granted Accreditation with type I recommendations, including a "special type I recommendation" for insufficient track record of compliance. This accreditation decision reflects the preliminary nature of the assessed performance. At a minimum, the recommendations will relate to limited or absent track records of performance in the functional areas where these are required. The effective date of the accreditation decision is the day after the *first* survey.

Early Survey Policy Options

Option 1

First survey

Can be conducted up to two months before operations begin. Survey of a limited set of standards addressing physical plant, policies and procedures, plans, and related structural considerations for individual care.

Successful outcome:
Provisional accreditation.

Second survey

Full survey conducted approximately six months after the first survey.

Possible outcomes:
Change in provisional accreditation status to accreditation with commendation, accreditation with or without type I recommendations, conditional accreditation, or preliminary nonaccreditation. The effective date of the accreditation decision is the day after the *second* survey.

Option 2

First survey

Must be in operation at least one month and has demonstrated a defined minimum level of individual care service with at least one individual in active treatment at the time of survey.

Possible outcomes:
Accreditation with type I recommendations, including a "special type I recommendation" for insufficient track record of compliance; conditional accreditation; or preliminary nonaccreditation.

Second survey

Conducted four months after the first survey. Survey addresses track record requirements not evaluated during the initial survey and may address standards compliance issues identified in the first survey. Based on the findings of either survey, follow-up activities such as focused surveys and written progress reports might be required.

Possible outcomes:
Accreditation with or without type I recommendations, conditional accreditation, or preliminary nonaccreditation. The effective date of the accreditation decision is the day after the *first* survey.

C. *The Second Survey.* The organization will undergo a follow-up survey in four months to address track record requirements that could not be assessed during the first survey due to the limited time of operation. The full scope of applicable standards will be reviewed with particular attention being paid to the issue of sustained performance since the first survey. Other follow-up activities such as focused surveys and written progress reports may be required on the basis of survey findings from either of the two surveys.

Initial Surveys

Organizations that are not currently accredited and that are seeking accreditation are eligible for an Initial Survey. The full scope of applicable standards will be reviewed during the survey. The scoring of the standards will be based on a 4-month track record of compliance, rather than the 12-month track record of compliance required for triennial surveys.

Sentinel Events

A sentinel event is an unexpected occurrence involving death or serious physical or psychological injury, or the risk thereof. Serious injury specifically includes loss of limb or function. The phrase, "or the risk thereof," includes any process variation for which a recurrence would carry a significant chance of a serious adverse outcome.

Such events are called "sentinel" because they signal the need for immediate investigation and response. Accredited organizations are expected to identify and respond appropriately to *all* sentinel events occurring in the organization or associated with services that the organization provides or provides for. Appropriate response includes a thorough and credible root cause analysis, implementation of improvements to reduce risk, and monitoring of the effectiveness of those improvements. An organization that completes an acceptable root cause analysis in response to a sentinel event will *not* be placed on Accreditation Watch.*

Organizations' activities in response to sentinel events will be routinely assessed as part of all triennial and random unannounced surveys.

Reporting of Sentinel Events to the Joint Commission

Organizations are encouraged to report a sentinel event to the Joint Commission if the event has resulted in an unanticipated death or major permanent loss of function,[†] not related to the natural course of the individual's illness or underlying condition,[‡] or the event is one of the following (even if the outcome was not death or major permanent loss of function):

- Suicide of an individual in a setting where the individual receives around-the-clock care (such as a hospital, residential treatment center, crisis stabilization center);
- Infant abduction or discharge to the wrong family;
- Rape;[§]
- Hemolytic transfusion reaction involving administration of blood or blood products having major blood group incompatibilities; or

---

* **Accreditation Watch** An attribute of an organization's Joint Commission accreditation status. A health care organization is placed on Accreditation Watch when a sentinel event has occurred and a thorough and credible root cause analysis of the sentinel event has not been completed within a specified time frame. Although Accreditation Watch status is not an official accreditation category, it can be publicly disclosed by the Joint Commission.

[†] "Major permanent loss of function" means sensory, motor, physiologic, or intellectual impairment not present on admission requiring continued treatment or life-style change. When major permanent loss of function cannot be immediately determined, reporting is not expected until either the individual is discharged with continued major loss of function, or two weeks have elapsed with persistent major loss of function, whichever occurs first.

[‡] A distinction is made between an adverse outcome that is related to the natural course of the individual's illness or underlying condition (not reportable) and a death or major permanent loss of function that is associated with the treatment, or lack of treatment, of that condition (reportable).

[§] The determination of "rape" is to be based on the health care organization's definition, consistent with applicable law and regulation. Reporting of an allegation of rape is not expected. The five-day time frame for reporting begins when a determination is made that a rape has occurred. Reporting of a rape is not expected where such reporting is prohibited by law.

- Surgery on the wrong individual or wrong body part.*

An organization that reports a sentinel event to the Joint Commission within five business days of its occurrence (or its discovery by the organization) and submits to the Joint Commission an acceptable root cause analysis (as described below) within 45 days of reporting the event, will *not* be placed on Accreditation Watch.

If the Joint Commission receives an inquiry about the accreditation status of the organization during the 45-day analysis period, the organization's accreditation status will be reported in the usual manner without reference to the sentinel event. If the inquirer specifically references the sentinel event, the Joint Commission will acknowledge that it is aware of the event and is working with the organization through the *sentinel event review process*.

An organization which experiences a sentinel event that does *not* meet the criteria for review under the Sentinel Event Policy is expected to complete a root cause analysis. However, the root cause analysis need *not* to be made available to the Joint Commission.

Figure 1 on page 14 is a flowchart depicting the sentinel event process and Table 1 on pages 15 through 18 details the steps taken during this process by both the Joint Commission and an organization experiencing a sentinel event.

Information Accuracy and Truthfulness Policy

Information provided at any time during the accreditation cycle by the organization and used by the Joint Commission for accreditation purposes must be accurate and truthful.† Such information may

- be provided verbally;
- be obtained through direct observation by Joint Commission surveyors;
- be derived from documents supplied by the organization to the Joint Commission; or
- involve data transmitted electronically to the Joint Commission.

The Joint Commission requires each organization seeking accreditation to engage in the accreditation process in good faith. The Joint Commission may deny or remove accreditation from any organization failing to participate in good faith by falsifying information presented in the accreditation process, among other possible acts.

The Joint Commission's information policy includes the following:

1. An organization must never provide the Joint Commission with falsified information during the accreditation process. The Joint Commission construes any efforts to do so as a violation of the organization's obligation to engage in the accreditation process in good faith.
2. Falsification is defined for this policy as the fabrication, in whole or in part, of any information provided by an applicant or accredited organization to the Joint Commission. This includes, but is not limited to, any redrafting, reformatting, or content deletion of documents.
3. The organization may submit additional material that summarizes or otherwise explains original information submitted to the Joint Commission. These materials must be properly identified, dated, and accompanied by the original documents.
4. Annually, each organization must submit to the Joint Commission a signed certification attesting to the accuracy and truthfulness of all information provided, or to be provided, throughout the accreditation cycle. Such certification should be signed by the CEO, the chairperson of the governing body, and the chief of the medical staff (or leader of the professional staff).

---

* All events of surgery on the wrong individual or wrong body part are reportable, regardless of the magnitude of the procedure.

† See Requirement 9 on page 44 in the Accreditation Participation Requirements chapter.

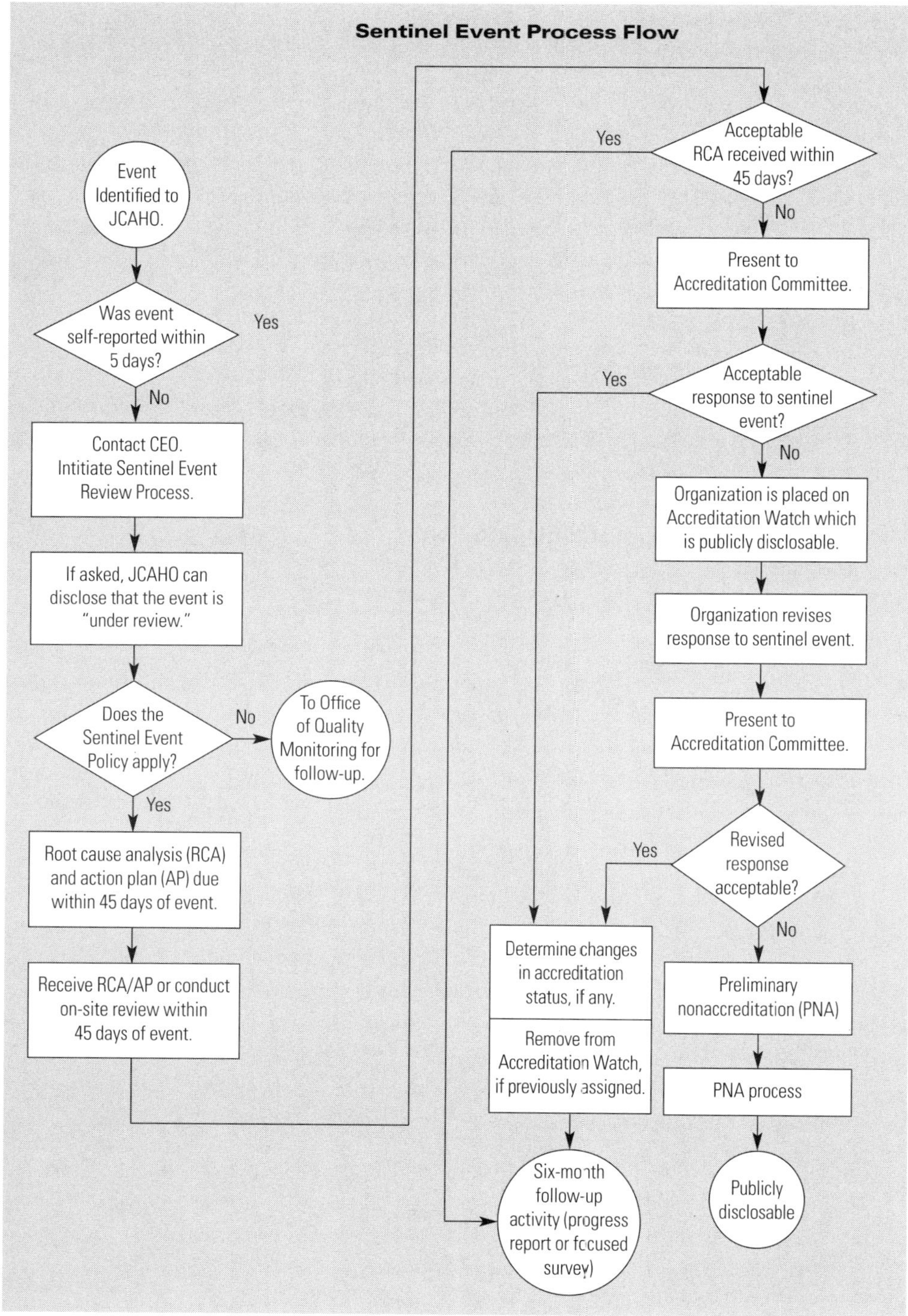

Figure 1. *This flowchart represents the Sentinel Event process.*

Table 1. Sentinel Event Process

Voluntary Self-Reporting of Sentinel Events to the Joint Commission

- If an organization wishes to self-report an occurrence in the subset of sentinel events that are subject to review by the Joint Commission, the organization will be required to complete a self-reporting form. To be considered a "self-reported sentinel event," this form must be received by the Joint Commission no later than five business days following the event, or the organization's becoming aware of the event.
- The organization will be required to
  - prepare an acceptable root cause analysis and action plan within 45 calendar days of the self-report, and
  - submit those documents to the Joint Commission, or otherwise provide for Joint Commission evaluation of its response to the sentinel event under an approved protocol, within 45 calendar days of the self-report.

Sentinel Events That Are Not Self-Reported

- If the Joint Commission becomes aware of a sentinel event subject to review under the Sentinel Event Policy that was not self-reported by the organization, the chief executive officer of the organization is contacted, and a preliminary assessment of the sentinel event is made.
- The organization will be required to
  - prepare an acceptable root cause analysis and action plan within 45 calendar days of the event, or of its becoming aware of the event, and
  - submit those documents to the Joint Commission, or otherwise provide for Joint Commission evaluation of its response to the sentinel event under an approved protocol, within 45 calendar days of the event, or of its becoming aware of the event.

On-site Review of a Sentinel Event

- An on-site review of a sentinel event will usually not be conducted unless it is determined that there is a potential ongoing threat to individual health or safety or potentially significant non-compliance with major Joint Commission standards. If an on-site ("for-cause") review is conducted, the organization will be billed an appropriate amount to cover the costs of conducting such a survey.

Disclosable Information

- If, during the 45-day analysis period, the Joint Commission receives an inquiry about the accreditation status of an organization that has experienced a sentinel event, the organization's accreditation status will be reported in the usual manner without making reference to the sentinel event.
- If the inquirer specifically references the sentinel event, the Joint Commission will acknowledge that it is aware of the event and is working with the organization through the *sentinel event review process*.

Initiation of Accreditation Watch

- If an organization has experienced a sentinel event but fails to submit or otherwise make available an acceptable root cause analysis and action plan, or otherwise provide for Joint Commission evaluation of its response to the sentinel event under an

continued on next page

Table 1. Sentinel Event Process (continued)

approved protocol, within 45 days of the event, or of its becoming aware of the event, a recommendation will be made to the Accreditation Committee to place the organization on Accreditation Watch. If the Accreditation Committee places the organization on Accreditation Watch, the organization will then be permitted an additional 15 days to submit an acceptable root cause analysis and action plan, or otherwise provide for Joint Commission evaluation of its response to the sentinel event under an approved protocol.

- The Accreditation Watch status will be publicly disclosed, and the organization will be offered assistance in performing a root cause analysis of the event.
- In all cases of organization refusal to permit review of information regarding a sentinel event in accordance with the Sentinel Event Policy and its approved protocols, the initial response by the Joint Commission is assignment of Accreditation Watch. Continued refusal may result in loss of accreditation.

The Organization's Response

Any organization that experiences a sentinel event subject to the Sentinel Event Policy must:

- Execute a root cause analysis that
  - focuses primarily on systems and processes, not individual performance;
  - progresses from special causes in clinical processes to common causes in organizational processes; and
  - identifies potential improvement in processes or systems that would tend to decrease the likelihood of such events in the future, or determines, after analysis, that no such improvement opportunities exist.
- Develop an action plan that is
  - based on the root cause analysis; and
  - as appropriate, identifies changes to be made in systems and processes—either through redesign or development of new systems or processes—that would reduce the risk of such events occurring in the future.
- Implement (after initial testing, if appropriate) the system and process improvements identified in its action plan.
- Design and apply an appropriate approach for evaluating the effectiveness of the improvements.

Submission of Root Cause Analysis and Action Plan

- The organization that experiences a sentinel event subject to the Sentinel Event Policy is asked to submit two documents:
  - the complete root cause analysis, including its findings; and
  - the resulting action plan that describes the organization's risk reduction strategies and strategy for evaluating their effectiveness.
- The root cause analysis and action plan are *not* to include the individual's name or the names of care givers involved in the sentinel event.
- Alternatively, if the organization has concerns about increased risk of legal exposure as a result of sending the root cause analysis documents to the Joint Commission, three additional options for on-site review are available:

continued on next page

Table 1. Sentinel Event Process (continued)

1. An on-site visit by a specially trained surveyor to review the root cause analysis and action plan, at a charge sufficient to cover the direct costs of the visit.
2. An on-site visit by a specially trained surveyor to conduct interviews and review relevant documentation to verify the appropriate response to the sentinel event, at a charge sufficient to cover the direct costs of the visit. For purposes of this review activity, "relevant documentation" includes, at a minimum, any documentation relevant to the organization's *process* for responding to sentinel events, and the action plan resulting from the analysis of the subject sentinel event (to serve as the basis for appropriate follow-up activity).
3. Where the organization meets specified criteria respecting the risk of waiving legal protection for root cause analysis information shared with the Joint Commission, an on-site visit by a specially trained surveyor to conduct interviews and review relevant documentation to obtain information about:
   - the process the organization uses in responding to sentinel events, and
   - the relevant policies and procedures preceding and following the organization's review of the specific event, and the implementation thereof,

   sufficient to permit inferences about the adequacy of the organization's response to the sentinel event, at a charge sufficient to cover the direct costs of the visit.

- A request for on-site option 1, 2, or 3 must be received by the Joint Commission at least 15 days prior to the due date for the root cause analysis and action plan.

The Joint Commission's Response

- Staff assesses the acceptability of the organization's response to the sentinel event, including the thoroughness and credibility of any root cause analysis information reviewed and the organization's action plan, and brings a recommendation to the Accreditation Committee at its next meeting following the due date for the organization's response.
- If the response is unacceptable, the organization is required to address the inadequacies and submit, or make available for review, a new root cause analysis and action plan, or otherwise provide for further Joint Commission evaluation of its response to the sentinel event, within 15 days of notification that the Accreditation Committee has found the response to be unacceptable.
- Depending on the nature and extent of the inadequacies of the organization's initial response to the sentinel event, the Joint Commission will determine whether an on-site visit should be made to assist the organization in understanding how to conduct an appropriate root cause analysis and develop an action plan.
- If on review, the organization's response is still not acceptable, or the organization fails to respond, staff will recommend to the Accreditation Committee that the organization be placed in Preliminary Nonaccreditation. If approved by the Accreditation Committee, this accreditation decision would be publicly disclosed, and the process for resolution of Preliminary Nonaccreditation would be initiated.
- When the organization's response (initial or revised) is found to be acceptable, the Joint Commission issues an *Official Accreditation Decision Report* which

continued on next page

Table 1. Sentinel Event Process (continued)

- reflects the Accreditation Committee's determination to continue or modify the organization's current accreditation status and terminate the Accreditation Watch (if previously assigned), and
- assigns an appropriate follow-up activity, typically a written progress report or follow-up visit to be conducted within six months.

Follow-up Activities

- The follow-up activity will assess, based on applicable standards, the implementation of system and process improvements identified in the action plan, the means by which the organization will continue to assess the effectiveness of those efforts, and the resolution of any type I recommendations. The follow-up activity will be conducted when the organization believes it can demonstrate effective implementation, but no later than six months following receipt of the *Official Accreditation Decision Report.*
- A decision to maintain or change the organization's accreditation status as a result of the follow-up activity or to assign additional follow-up requirements will be based on existing decision rules unless otherwise determined by the Accreditation Committee.
- Each sentinel event evaluated under the Joint Commission's Sentinel Event Policy will be reviewed at the organization's next full accreditation survey. This review will focus on implementation of risk reduction strategies and the effectiveness of these actions.

Handling Sentinel Event-Related Documents

- Upon completing the review of any submitted root cause analysis and action plan and abstracting the required data elements for the Joint Commission's Sentinel Event Database, the original root cause analysis documents will be returned to the organization and any copies will be shredded. Handling of these sensitive documents is restricted to specially trained staff in accordance with procedures designed to protect the confidentiality of the documents. The action plan resulting from the analysis of the sentinel event will be retained to serve as the basis for the follow-up activity.
- Once the action plan has been implemented to the satisfaction of the Joint Commission, as determined through follow-up activities, the Joint Commission will return the action plan to the organization.

5. The Joint Commission does not release the organization's accreditation award or survey report until it has received the organization's properly signed certification for the current year.
6. The Joint Commission conducts an evaluation when it has cause to believe that an accredited organization may have provided falsified information. Except as otherwise authorized by the president of the Joint Commission, the evaluation includes an unannounced on-site survey. This survey uses special protocols designed to address the alleged information falsification. It assesses the degree of actual organization compliance with the standards and their intent statements that are the subject of the allegation, if appropriate.

7. The Joint Commission immediately takes action to deny accreditation or remove the accreditation award from an accredited organization whenever the Joint Commission is reasonably persuaded that the organization has provided falsified information.
8. The Joint Commission notifies responsible federal and state government agencies of any organization subject to such action.
9. If an organization becomes not accredited because it provided falsified information, the Joint Commission prohibits it from participating in the accreditation process for a period of one year. The president of the Joint Commission, for good cause only, may waive all or a portion of this waiting period.

Public Information Policy

The Joint Commission is committed to making relevant and accurate information about surveyed health care organizations available to interested persons. Information regarding the performance of a health care organization not only assists providers in improving their services, but also helps educate consumers. It also may help consumers and purchasers make informed choices in selecting health care providers. At the same time, it is important that confidentiality be maintained for certain information to encourage candor in the accreditation process. This candor facilitates improvement of the quality of health care to the benefit of the public.

Performance Reports. Performance reports are designed to provide useful and understandable information about the performance of organizations accredited by the Joint Commission. The Joint Commission began releasing organization-specific performance reports in December 1994 for most types of health care organizations undergoing full surveys after January 1, 1994. Reports for laboratories subsequently became available for those labs surveyed after January 1, 1995. Reports for health care networks will become available once this accreditation program includes a statistically significant sample. Joint Commission performance reports for each accredited organization include the following information:

- The date of the most recent triennial survey;
- The accreditation decision based on the most recent triennial survey;
- An organization's current accreditation status, including any designation attached to that status, such as Accreditation Watch, and the date on which that designation became effective;
- The date of the most recent follow-up activity for the organization, if any;
- The organization's overall evaluation score, based on the triennial survey, and national comparison to scores for comparable organizations;
- The organization's score for each performance area evaluated and national comparisons to scores for comparable organizations;
- Performance areas with recommendations for improvement;
- Subsequent change(s) in accreditation status, if any;
- Subsequent resolution of recommendations for improvement and the date(s) of resolution for specific performance areas;
- Subsequent new performance area(s) having recommendations for improvement and the date(s) assigned;
- The organization's updated overall evaluation score and performance area scores; and
- Organizational and operational components included in the accreditation survey.

Each accredited organization is afforded the opportunity to prepare a commentary of up to two pages regarding its performance report. The commentary is to accompany any organization performance reports distributed by the Joint Commission.

Each performance report released by the Joint Commission is also to be accompanied by an explanatory document that supports the accurate interpretation of the report.

The Joint Commission also may provide access to performance reports through the Internet and may make available information contained in performance reports to other third-party providers of information.

Performance measurement data will be included in performance reports when those data become an integral part of the accreditation process. These data will be released provided that the following conditions are met:

- The data are accompanied by an explanation of their
  - source or derivation;
  - accuracy, reliability, and validity;
  - appropriate uses; and
  - limitations and potential misuses.
- No data will be published unless it contains at least 12 monthly data points.
- No data will be published until the organization has had an opportunity to comment on them.

Information That is Publicly Disclosed on Request. In addition to information provided in performance reports, the following information may be obtained by writing or calling the Joint Commission:

- The organization's accreditation history;
- Any special recognition conferred on the organization, such as the Ernest A. Codman Award or participation in ORYX PLUS;
- Survey fees paid by an accredited organization;
- The organization's scheduled survey date(s) once the organization has been notified of the dates;
- Confirmation of the occurrence of a sentinel event in an accredited organization and the Joint Commission's intent to evaluate this occurrence;
- Applicable standards used for an accreditation survey;
- For a tailored survey, the organizational component(s) contributing to a conditional accreditation or denial of accreditation decision;
- Whether there were any type I recommendations for which the Joint Commission had no, or insufficient, evidence of resolution when an organization withdrew from accreditation;
- The performance areas for which the Joint Commission had no, or insufficient, evidence of resolution of type I recommendations when an organization withdrew from accreditation; and
- Whether an on-site evaluation of an organization in which a sentinel event has occurred is to be or has been conducted.

Public Release of Complaint Information. The Joint Commission responds to complaints received about accredited organizations. Complaints may be forwarded by HCFA or other federal or state agencies having oversight responsibilities for health care organizations, or may be received directly from consumers, payers, or health care professionals. The Joint Commission addresses all complaints that pertain to quality of care issues within the scope of Joint Commission standards.

The Joint Commission releases the following information relating to complaints about accredited organizations upon request:

- The applicable standards areas involved in a Joint Commission complaint review;
- Since the last triennial survey, the
  - number of written complaints filed against an accredited organization,
  - number of complaints investigated by the Joint Commission, and
  - performance areas in which type I recommendations were issued as a result of complaint evaluation activities; and

- When an unannounced or unscheduled survey is based on information derived from a complaint or public sources, the nature of the complaint or information upon which the survey is based.

The Joint Commission also provides the following information to complainants regarding their complaints:

- The course of action to be taken regarding the complaint.
- Whether the Joint Commission has decided to take action regarding an organization's accreditation status following completion of the complaint investigation:
  - If the Joint Commission has decided to take no action, the complainant is to be so advised.
  - If the Joint Commission has taken action, the complainant is to be advised in conformance with the guidelines for release of complaint information as set forth above.

Release of Aggregate Performance Data. The Joint Commission reserves the right to publish or release aggregate performance data.

Confidential Information. The Joint Commission keeps confidential the following information received or developed during the accreditation process:

- Information relating to compliance with specific accreditation standards obtained from an organization before, during, or following the accreditation survey;
- The content of an organization's root cause analysis prepared in response to a sentinel event or in response to other circumstances specified by the Joint Commission;
- All other materials that may contribute to the accreditation decision (for example, survey report forms, medical records);
- Written staff analyses and Accreditation Committee minutes and agenda materials; and
- The *Official Accreditation Decision Report.*

This policy applies to all organizations with an accreditation history, except as provided below or by law, or as authorized by responsible organization officials.

*Data Release to Government Agencies.** The Joint Commission provides federal, state, or local government agencies specific accreditation-related information under the following circumstances:

- When the Joint Commission identifies a serious situation in an organization that may jeopardize the safety of individuals or the public; and
- When an organization, certified for participation in a federal or state program or licensed to operate on the basis of its accreditation, is assigned a conditional accreditation, preliminary nonaccreditation, or not accredited decision. The Joint Commission so advises the organization's CEO and provides timely notice to local, state, and federal authorities having jurisdiction. The information provided to government agencies includes
  - the accreditation decision, including any designation attached to that status, such as Accreditation Watch;
  - all type I recommendations;
  - a statement, if any, provided by the organization regarding the validity of the Joint Commission survey finding; and

* Section 92, PL 96-499, the Omnibus Budget Reconciliation Act of 1980, requires that Medicare providers include, in all their contracts for services costing $10,000 or more in any 12-month period, a clause allowing the Secretary of the U.S. Department of Health and Human Services (DHHS), the U.S. Comptroller General, or their representatives to examine the contract and the contractor's books and records. The Joint Commission herein stipulates that if its charges to any such organization amount to $10,000 or more in any 12-month period, the contract or any agreement on which such charges are based and any of the Joint Commission's books, documents, and records that may be necessary to verify the extent and nature of Joint Commission costs will be available to the Secretary of DHHS, the Comptroller General, or any of their duly authorized representatives for four years after the survey. The same conditions will apply to any subcontracts the Joint Commission has with related organizations if the payments under such contracts amount to $10,000 or more in any 12-month period.

- ❑ for conditionally accredited organizations, a copy of the approved plan of correction and the results of the plan of correction follow-up survey.

Joint Commission Right to Clarify. The Joint Commission reserves the right to clarify information, even if the information involved would otherwise be considered confidential, when an organization disseminates inaccurate information regarding its accreditation.

Performance Reports

The performance report provides summary information about an organization's performance on current Joint Commission standards relating to quality of care and service. Performance reports are created at the organization level and provide comparative accreditation information gathered from similar organizations surveyed nationwide. A performance report includes such information as

- the organization's accreditation decision;
- a listing of the areas having specific recommendations for improvement;
- performance area scores (with national comparative data); and
- an overall evaluation score (with national comparative data).

Results of follow-up activities are also reported on the performance report, including current information regarding

- the organization's accreditation status;
- performance area scores; and
- the remaining performance areas that have recommendations for improvement.

A performance report is created once an organization's accreditation decision is final. If an organization requests a revision to its *Official Accreditation Decision Report* or its survey report, the Joint Commission *will not* release the organization's performance report until the revision is addressed.

On receipt, an organization has 30 days to submit a Two-Page Commentary on the performance report. The commentary is optional. The Joint Commission sends the performance report, an explanatory document, and the organization's commentary to individuals requesting the organization's performance report. The Joint Commission sends *only* the performance report and the explanatory document if an organization chooses not to prepare a commentary. The performance report is available to the public 30 days after its receipt by the organization.

Survey Fees

The Joint Commission determines survey fees annually as needed to maintain the cost of its operations. Surveyed organizations are charged for all surveys with the exception of focused surveys and random unannounced surveys. The Joint Commission bases an organization's survey fees on several factors, including the volume and type of services provided, and the survey's length and location. An organization may request a longer survey, but a fee will be charged for the additional time. Such requests should be sent to the organization's accreditation service specialist. Contact the Pricing Unit at the Joint Commission at 630/792-5665 for a fee schedule or more information on survey fees.

The Joint Commission sends an invoice when it schedules an organization for survey. It asks the organization to pay the fees according to specified terms. The Joint Commission charges an organization the fee rate in effect at the time of survey. For an initial survey, an organization must send a nonrefundable processing fee with the Application for Survey. The Joint Commission credits this payment toward the organization's total fee.

The Joint Commission offers organizations two payment options. An organization can either

- pay the full survey fee when billed or
- spread the payments over a three and one-half-month period.

Under the second option, an organization must pay one-half of the full survey fee at the time of billing (about six weeks before the survey date) and the balance no later than 60 days after the survey date.

An organization *that did not pay* its survey fee in full prior to issuance of the accreditation decision and report must remit the outstanding balance within 60 days from receipt of the report. Failure to provide timely payment may result in the loss of accreditation. The Joint Commission notifies an organization with significant standards compliance problems of either a conditional accreditation or a preliminary nonaccreditation decision as soon as possible, whether or not payment has been received.

Before the Survey

An organization seeking to undergo the accreditation process for the first time will want to read this section. It provides information on the steps leading to a full accreditation survey. These include the application process, the assignment of an accreditation service specialist, survey scheduling, the assignment of a survey team, the development of a survey agenda, public notification of the survey, and the conduct of a public information interview.

An organization seeking to renew its accreditation may wish to review selected information, including the description of the application for resurvey process, policies regarding survey scheduling, postponements, and delays, the notification of the public about a forthcoming Joint Commission survey, and the conduct of a public information interview.

Application for Survey

An organization begins the accreditation process by completing an Application for Survey. This document provides essential information about an organization, including ownership, demographics, and types and volume of services provided.

The Application for Survey

- describes the organization seeking accreditation;
- requires the organization to provide the Joint Commission with all official records and reports of public or publicly recognized licensing (for example, a state license), examining, reviewing, or planning bodies;*
- authorizes the Joint Commission to obtain any records and reports not possessed by the organization; and
- when accepted, establishes the terms of the relationship between the organization and the Joint Commission.

An organization may request an Application for Survey by writing to

Joint Commission on Accreditation of Healthcare Organizations
Packaging Unit
One Renaissance Boulevard
Oakbrook Terrace, IL 60181

or by calling 630/792-5519.

The Joint Commission sends an application for resurvey to accredited organizations approximately six months before the due date of their next triennial survey. Organizations that have not received an Application for Survey four months before their due date should call the Joint Commission at the number listed above. The Joint Commission will notify the organization of the scheduled survey at least four weeks before the survey date.

* See Requirement 1 on page 40 in the Accreditation Participation Requirements chapter.

Accuracy of the Application Information. The Joint Commission schedules surveys based on information provided in the organization's Application for Survey. With the information provided, the Joint Commission determines the number of days required for a survey and the composition of the survey team.

Inaccurate information in the Application for Survey may necessitate an additional survey, which could delay the Joint Commission's accreditation decision and survey report. The organization may also incur additional survey charges.

*Handling Changes During the Application Process.** The organization must notify the Joint Commission immediately if it undergoes a change that modifies the information reported in the Application for Survey. Information that must be reported includes

- a change in ownership;
- a change in location;
- a significant increase or decrease in the volume of services;
- the addition of a new type of health service; or
- the deletion of an existing health service or site of care.

The Joint Commission may schedule an additional survey for a later date if its surveyor or survey team arrives at the organization and discovers that a change was not reported. The Joint Commission may also survey any *unreported* services addressed by its standards. The Joint Commission will make the final accreditation decision for the organization only after surveying *all* services provided by the organization for which the Joint Commission has standards. Information reported in the Application for Survey is bound by the Joint Commission's policy on information accuracy and truthfulness (see pages 13, 18–19).

Survey Scheduling and Postponements

Schedules for Surveys. The Joint Commission schedules surveys systematically and efficiently to keep survey fees to a minimum. Therefore, organizations are encouraged to accept scheduled survey dates. Resurveys are scheduled within 45 days before or after the organizations triennial due date. An organization's first full accreditation survey, an initial survey, must be scheduled within one year from the time the Joint Commission receives the organization's application.

Special Requests. The Joint Commission tries to honor written requests specifying dates during which an organization prefers not to be surveyed. The organization should make the request with the completed Application for Survey, whenever possible. However, circumstances may prevent the Joint Commission from accommodating these requests.

Definition of Postponement. Under limited circumstances, the Joint Commission can provide for the postponement of surveys beyond the 45-day window. A *postponement* is an organization's request to alter an already scheduled survey date or to alter the survey date before it is actually scheduled. An organization should direct a request for a postponement to its accreditation service specialist.

Survey Postponement Policy. A request to postpone a survey may be granted if one or more of the following criteria are met:

- a natural disaster or other major unforeseen event has occurred that has totally or substantially disrupted operations;
- the organization is involved in a major strike, has ceased admitting individuals, and is transferring individuals to other facilities or organizations;
- individuals and/or the organization are being moved to a new building on the day or days of the survey; or

---

* See Requirement 2 on page 40 in the Accreditation Participation Requirements chapter.

- the Joint Commission has provided less than four weeks advance notice to the organization (by telephone or in writing) of the survey date(s).

Note: *If a survey postponement is requested because of a natural disaster, strike, or movement to a new building, an on-site extension survey may be required if the organization is continuing to provide individual care services.*

If one or more of the listed criteria are met, a survey may be postponed for up to six months from the anniversary or due date. If the postponement or delay is to be more than six months and the organization is accredited, an on-site extension survey will normally be conducted.

An organization undergoing its first Joint Commission survey will be required to specify on its application for survey the month in which it wishes to be surveyed. Following the scheduling of the survey, the organization would *only* be permitted to postpone its survey if it meets the above criteria.

Fees for Postponements. The Joint Commission may, at its option, approve a survey postponement for an organization not meeting any of the criteria described above. In such cases, the organization is charged a fee to defray costs and may be required to undergo an extension survey. The Joint Commission will charge the base fee for the survey of each program being postponed. The Joint Commission reserves the right, however, to deny any request for a postponement, regardless of the organization's willingness to pay the special fee.

Timeliness of Application and Deposits. The Joint Commission requires an organization to submit a new Application for Survey if the organization does not accept a scheduled survey within one year. This ensures that the organization's information is current.

A nonrefundable, nontransferable survey deposit is required for initial surveys only. The Joint Commission applies the deposit to the organization's survey fee if a survey is conducted.

Forfeiture of Survey Deposit. An organization scheduled for an initial survey will forfeit its survey deposit if its survey is not conducted within 12 months of submission of its application. The organization must then reapply and submit a new survey deposit to begin the accreditation process again.

The Survey Agenda

The Joint Commission's accreditation service specialist works with the organization to develop a tentative survey agenda based on survey task assignments required as part of the survey. A generic agenda template will be sent to all organizations with a similar number of required survey days and similar survey teams. The draft of the tentative agenda is reviewed and revisions made, as appropriate.

The organization and its accreditation service specialist collaboratively develop the final agenda used for the accreditation survey. A planning questionnaire is sent to the organization approximately six months before the organization's due date for survey to facilitate this process. The questionnaire solicits information about

- the organization's individual care settings including inpatient, ambulatory/outpatient, special care, imaging, and anesthetizing units or locations, and
- optional survey activities the organization may wish to have included in the survey.

The Joint Commission provides other materials to assist the organization in identifying

- staff that should be involved in various survey activities, and
- documents that should be available to the surveyors during the on-site survey.

The final agenda reflects survey activities and the staff and documents required during the survey.

Notifying the Public About a Joint Commission Survey

The Joint Commission evaluates all relevant information about an organization's compliance with applicable standards. It therefore requires a surveyed organization to inform the public of a scheduled full survey and invite them to provide the surveyor or survey team with relevant information.* The organization must provide an opportunity for members of the public to participate in a public information interview during a full survey, including both surveys under Option 2 of the Early Survey Policy (see pages 10–11). A full survey refers to the survey of all components of an organization under all applicable standards. The public includes, but is not limited to

- individuals and their families;
- personal advocates and advocacy groups;
- members of the community for whom services are provided; and
- personnel and staff.

Public Posting. The surveyed organization is responsible for making the public information interview process widely known and effective as a source of compliance information in the accreditation process. The Joint Commission requires an organization scheduled for full survey to post announcements of

- the survey date,
- the opportunity for a public information interview, and
- how to request an interview.

In the event that all organization components are not surveyed at the same time, the posting requirement applies at the time the primary program is surveyed. For example, if an organization with organization, long term care, and home care components is scheduled for a tailored survey in which the organization is the primary program and each component's survey is scheduled for a different date, the notice of survey is to be posted consistent with the organization's survey dates.

To maximize participation, postings must be made throughout the organization, including components being surveyed at a different time, in the form provided by the Joint Commission. See Figure 3, above, for an example of a Public Notice form. This example may be used by the organization, or the organization may design its own Public Notice form that conveys the same information as this example. An organization should post notices in staff eating areas, break rooms, on bulletin boards near major entrances, and in treatment or residential areas. In addition, the organization must provide each staff person with a written announcement of the survey, if such postings are not likely to be seen by all staff.

Advance Notice. The Joint Commission requires an organization scheduled for survey to post public notices at least 30 days before the scheduled date. An organization receiving the scheduled date less than 30 days before the survey date should post public notices promptly. Notices must remain posted until the survey is completed.

Informing the Community. The organization must take reasonable steps to inform its community of the opportunity for public information interviews during the full survey at least 30 days before the survey. Steps include

- informing all advocacy groups (such as organized individual groups and unions) that have substantively communicated with it in the previous 12 months;
- reaching other members of the community through means such as a public service announcement on radio or television, a classified advertisement in a local newspaper, or a notice in a community newsletter or other publication;* and
- informing individuals who inquire about the survey of the survey date(s) and opportunity to participate.

---

* See Requirement 7 on page 43 in the Accreditation Participation Requirements chapter.

Compliance with the Public Information Interview Policy. The surveyor(s) reviews the organization's compliance with the policy outlined above. The team indicates at the exit conference whether it believes the organization has complied with the policy and reports on this to the Joint Commission. An initial failure to comply with the public information interview policy ordinarily results in a type I recommendation (see "Accreditation Decision" on page 31). As a result, the Joint Commission may also conduct a postsurvey public information interview, if requested.

In addition, the surveyor(s) conducting a postsurvey public information interview also conduct(s) whatever follow-up survey he or she (they) believes appropriate in view of the information obtained during the public information interview. An organization's subsequent failure to comply with the Joint Commission's public information interview policy may result in loss or denial of its accreditation. A fee is associated with public information interviews conducted after the survey of an organization that is not in compliance with the public information interview policy.

Conduct of the Public Information Interview

*Handling Requests.** Individuals requesting a public information interview are to forward their requests and the nature of the information they will provide in writing to the Joint Commission. The organization must explain this process in its communications. To ensure participation, individuals are encouraged to forward written requests as soon as possible, and no later than five days before the scheduled survey.

Sometimes an individual may make a written request for a public information interview directly to the organization. When this occurs, the organization must promptly forward it to the Joint Commission. An organization receiving *oral requests* should instruct individuals to make the request in writing and mail them to the Joint Commission. The organization should provide individuals needing assistance in doing this with the necessary support.

Scheduling Interviews. The organization must provide potential public information interview participants with sufficient advance notice. The Joint Commission acknowledges all public information interview requests and provides the organization with copies of the acknowledgments. Prior to the survey, the Joint Commission schedules a time-limited public information interview to be conducted during the survey. The organization is responsible for notifying the individuals requesting public information interviews of the interview's exact date, time, and place. The organization must try to alleviate any potential concerns about reprisals to individuals who participate in the interview process.

Interview Eligibility. Individuals whose written requests arrive late or who simply appear at the stated time, requesting the opportunity to be heard without a prior written request, are heard by a Joint Commission surveyor if time permits. Otherwise, the surveyor informs them that it is not possible to honor their requests and then offers them the opportunity to provide a subsequent written statement.

Individuals contacting the Joint Commission and stating an interest in supplying information anonymously are informed that they may provide written complaints through the Joint Commission's complaint process. The Joint Commission will maintain confidentiality, as requested.

The Interview Process. The Joint Commission's survey team conducts the public information interview. A representative of the surveyed organization may attend, unless the individual requesting the public information interview asks that no representative from the organization be present. The Joint Commission will honor such requests. The interview will be conducted on the organization's premises, whether a representative from the organization is present or not. The organization is expected to provide reasonable accommodations for all public information interviews.

* See Requirement 8 on page 43 in the Accreditation Participation Requirements chapter.

An interview consists of the orderly receipt of information, orally or in writing, within a set time limit. The interview is *not* a debate between an organization's representative and an interviewee. Surveyors may, however, ask clarifying questions.

In addition, surveyors will not debate with or convey conclusions to any interviewee. Rather, the Joint Commission considers the information gathered by the survey team along with its findings and recommendations during the survey process.

During the Survey

This section includes information relevant to an organization that has applied for an accreditation survey and is ready for the survey process. It provides an overview of the survey process itself, the survey team and its leadership, and surrounding issues. These include how the Joint Commission handles findings of individual care or safety concerns, preliminary reports and how they are prepared, and the conduct of a leadership exit conference.

The Survey Process in Brief

Overview. During an accreditation survey, the Joint Commission evaluates an organization's performance of functions and processes aimed at continuously improving individual outcomes. The survey process focuses on assessing performance of important individual-centered and organization functions that support quality individual care. The process has moved away from evaluating specific departments and services. The survey team described below assesses an organization based on the performance-focused standards included in this manual. Surveys are designed to be individualized to each organization, to be consistent, and to support the organization's efforts to improve performance. Depending on the scope of the survey, organizations receive a 1-, 2-, or 3-day survey, conducted on a triennial basis.

Survey Team Composition. Accreditation surveys are conducted by one or more surveyors. The selection of the surveyor and number of surveyors assigned is based on the information provided in its Application for Survey. All surveyors assess and provide consultation regarding all functions addressed by the standards.

In addition, depending on the organization's service configuration, there may be a specialized surveyor addressing such areas as long term care, home care, or ambulatory medical care services. The findings of specialized surveyors are integrated into the organization's accreditation decision and survey report.

Survey Team Leadership. When a team is assigned, one of the experienced surveyors on each organization survey team is designated as the "team leader." The team leader is responsible for integration, coordination, and communication of on-site survey activities. In addition to direct participation as an active member of the survey team, the team leader serves as the primary point of on-site contact between the organization and the Joint Commission. Among other responsibilities, the team leader leads the opening conference and the daily and exit briefings.

Opening Conference and Performance Improvement Overview. After the organization has completed the presurvey steps described in pages 23 through 28, the first actual survey activity involves an opening conference. This conference lays the groundwork for the survey.

Following the opening conference, organization staff orient the survey team to the organization's approach to performance improvement. This is an opportunity for an organization to showcase its program to measure, assess, and improve its performance of the important functions addressed by the standards.

Document Review. After completing the opening conference and the performance improvement overview, the surveyors begin the assessment process by reviewing key documents that focus on the organization's performance. Documents include committee minutes, reports of performance-improvement activities, and measurement data. Certain bylaws, planning documents, and other evidence of performance also will be included.

Interviews with Organization Leaders. Interviews with the organization's leaders occur both early and at later stages in the survey process. Interviews address the collaboration of senior leaders in the performance improvement process and the roles played by administration, department directors, medical staff, and nursing leaders.

Visits to Individual Care and Service Settings or Program Settings. Visits to individual care settings play a major role in the organization survey process. Surveyors visit settings where individuals' needs are assessed or where individuals receive care. Settings include living sites and service program sites.

During these visits, the survey team interacts with managers, direct care providers—including members of the clinical staff, other organization staff, and individuals. The team also

- tours the setting to address environment of care, individual care, staff communication, individual rights issues, and infection control; and
- reviews open clinical records with a group of direct care providers.

Team members integrate their findings to assess compliance levels.

Function Interviews. These interviews gather a multidisciplinary group of the organization's staff who have important responsibilities related to a given function. They follow up on issues identified in the document review and reflect observations made by surveyors in visits to individual care settings.

Scoring Compliance Against Track Record Requirements. Accredited organizations are expected to remain in continuous compliance with the standards and their intent statements throughout the interval between surveys. However, for practical purposes in conducting the survey, surveyors will ordinarily limit their evaluation of the organization's track record of compliance. In addition to the performance expectations described in the scoring section of each functional chapter, and subject to exercise of appropriate discretion, organizations ordinarily will be expected to show a track record of compliance for one year before a triennial survey. Surveyors may evaluate compliance over a shorter or longer time frame depending on circumstances encountered during the survey. For example, the required time frame for full compliance with applicable standards and intents for new services will not exceed the time the service has been in operation. In another example, certain activities that are conducted infrequently, such as biennial credentialing, may require evaluation over a longer interval to ensure an adequate sample size for valid assessment.

For a triennial survey, an organization's track record generally will impact the scoring of standards according to the following matrix:

Score 1	12 months before survey
Score 2	9 to 11 months before survey
Score 3	6 to 8 months before survey
Score 4	5 months or less before survey
Score 5	No process in place

During initial or focused surveys, an organization's track record generally will impact the scoring of standards according to the following matrix:

Score 1	4 months before survey
Score 2	3 months before survey
Score 3	2 months before survey
Score 4	1 month before survey
Score 5	Less than 1 month before survey

Feedback Sessions. Final scores about compliance are not reached until all individual care settings have been visited and all other assessment interviews and activities have been conducted. However, surveyors will communicate their observations at daily briefings and during a medical staff luncheon, as requested by the organization.

Final On-Site Survey Activities. At the leadership exit conference, described on page 00, the survey team will present complete survey findings, a preliminary written report, and a potential accreditation decision.

Individual Care or Safety Concerns

The Joint Commission may consider for accreditation purposes a surveyor's finding that some aspect of an organization's operation is having or may have a direct, adverse effect on individual health or safety. The Joint Commission may obtain expert consultation regarding these findings.

Surveyors will notify the organization's CEO and Joint Commission corporate office staff immediately if they identify any condition they believe poses an immediate threat to public or individual safety. The president of the Joint Commission, or if the president is unavailable, a designated vice president, can then issue an expedited preliminary nonaccreditation decision based on such notification. He or she will promptly inform the organization's CEO and appropriate governmental authorities of this decision. The Accreditation Committee of the Board of Commissioners will confirm or reverse the decision at its next meeting.

Laptop Technology and Preliminary Reports

Use of Laptop Technology. Each day, after the survey team performs the activities described on pages 31 and 28–30, team members enter survey data and documentation on laptop computers. These computers are equipped with specially designed decision-support software. The software guides the accurate entry of findings, integrates the findings of multiple surveyors, and calculates standard-level scores, thereby allowing surveyors, as a team, to review the information and make necessary adjustments.

Presentation of a Preliminary Report. The survey team reviews the results of integrated individual findings. Then, with the use of laptop-based decision support software, the team produces a preliminary report on-site. Preliminary reports include the accreditation decision grid, preliminary type I and supplemental recommendations (as applicable), the projected outcome or potential accreditation decision, and any follow-up requirements. The findings of specialized, add-on surveyors are integrated as a part of the preliminary report.

The team leader meets with the organization's CEO prior to the leadership exit conference and provides him or her with a copy of the preliminary report. The CEO determines whether or not the preliminary report is distributed at the leadership exit conference. The survey team uses preliminary report contents in making its leadership exit conference presentations.

Use of the Preliminary Report. Recognizing that many organizations are eager to release the results of their accreditation survey immediately following the survey, it must be emphasized that this is a *preliminary* report, not a *final* decision. The final decision will be made following an appropriate review at the Joint Commission's central office. In some instances, a change will be made in the accreditation report. Therefore, organizations are encouraged to not make any formal announcement as a result of a preliminary report.

In choosing to publicize the preliminary report, organizations should state that the findings are preliminary. If the Joint Commission is contacted by members of the media or community we will not be able to confirm any accreditation decision because no such decision will have yet been made. Once the final report is sent to the organization, the accreditation decision is officially public.

Leadership Exit Conference

Joint Commission surveyors confer with the organization's CEO and other leaders* as part of a leadership exit conference for each survey. The purpose of the conference is to

- review the preliminary report, if the CEO determines it will be made available;
- gain agreement between the team and the organization regarding survey findings; and
- report to the organization the potential accreditation decision based on the findings.

The survey team leader presides during the conference. The team leader and the other surveyors present their findings on any significant standards compliance issues. In addition, they discuss underlying causes of the compliance issues and recommend improvements. Each member of the team presents findings by function. The surveyors provide the organization's representatives with an opportunity to clarify issues and respond to recommendations. The surveyors also confer on survey findings that may not be directly related to the standards, if requested.

Following the close of the leadership exit conference, the survey team will, as appropriate

- revise or include additional information from the conference in the team's report;
- identify, for the Joint Commission's central office staff, challenged findings that have not been resolved; and
- issue a new preliminary report, if needed.

After the Survey

This section includes information relevant to an organization that recently has participated in an accreditation survey. Material includes information on types of accreditation decisions, how to request revisions to the survey report, how to appeal "not accredited" decisions, and how to use and display an accreditation award.

Accreditation Decision

The Joint Commission provides the organization with an accreditation decision in its *Official Accreditation Decision Report*. This accreditation decision involves processing the surveyors' findings according to specific aggregation rules and decision rules established by the Accreditation Committee of the Board of Commissioners. The "Accreditation and Appeal Procedures" chapter outlines specific accreditation procedures.

There are seven possible accreditation decisions:

1. Accreditation with Commendation;
2. Accreditation;
3. Accreditation with Type I Recommendations;
4. Provisional Accreditation;
5. Conditional Accreditation;
6. Preliminary Nonaccreditation; and
7. Not Accredited.

Table 2 (pages 32–33) provides a description of each category and the conditions that lead to it.

An organization's wish to withdraw from the accreditation process after undergoing survey and before a final decision has been made does not terminate the decision-making process. The Joint Commission will reach a final accreditation decision.

---

* **leader** An individual who sets expectations, develops plans, and implements procedures to assess and improve the quality of the organization's governance, management, clinical, and support functions and processes. Leaders include at least members of the governing body; the chief executive officer and other senior managers; clinical leaders (clinical leaders include health care professionals with overall responsibility to plan, organize, and operate a clinical service or program and may include but are not limited to the clinical director, discipline chief, and unit or service director); and staff members in a leadership position within the organization.

Table 2. Types of Accreditation Decisions

Accreditation Decision Category	Conditions That Lead to this Type of Decision
Accreditation with Commendation	The highest accreditation decision that is awarded when an organization has demonstrated exemplary performance in complying with Joint Commission standards. An organization is eligible for accreditation with commendation (1) if the summary grid score for all applicable programs is 90 or higher; (2) if no type I recommendations have been assigned; and (3) if all applicable programs of the organization that are eligible for survey have been surveyed and each applicable program meets criteria 1 and 2 stated above.
Accreditation without Type I Recommendations	An accreditation decision that results when an organization has demonstrated acceptable compliance with Joint Commission standards in all performance areas.
Accreditation with Type I Recommendations	An accreditation decision that results when an organization receives at least one recommendation addressing insufficient or unsatisfactory standards compliance in a specific performance area or a "Special Type I Recommendation" (for example, a special type I recommendation assigned when a requirement in the "Accreditation Participation Requirements" chapter is not met). Resolution of type I recommendations must be achieved within stipulated time frames (through a focused survey or a written progress report submitted by the organization) to maintain accreditation.
Provisional Accreditation	An accreditation decision that results when an organization has demonstrated satisfactory compliance with the selected

continued on next page

Table 2. Types of Accreditation Decisions (continued)

Provisional Accreditation *(continued)*	standards applied during the organization's initial survey under the Early Survey Policy—Option 1. The second survey, or full survey, is conducted approximately six months later to allow the organization sufficient time to demonstrate a track record of performance and results in the organization's receiving one of the other official accreditation decisions.
Conditional Accreditation	An accreditation decision that results when an organization is not in substantial compliance with Joint Commission standards but is believed to be capable of achieving acceptable standards compliance within a stipulated time period. Findings of correction, which serve as the basis for further consideration of awarding full accreditation, must be demonstrated through a short-term follow-up survey.
Preliminary Nonaccreditation	An accreditation decision that is assigned to an organization when it is found to be in significant noncompliance with Joint Commission standards or when its accreditation is preliminarily withdrawn by the Joint Commission for other reasons (for example, falsification of documents) **prior** to the determination of the final decision (for example, Not Accredited). Preliminary nonaccreditation is an appealable accreditation decision.
Not Accredited	An accreditation decision that results when an organization is denied accreditation because of significant noncompliance with Joint Commission standards, when its accreditation is withdrawn by the Joint Commission for other reasons, or when the organization voluntarily withdraws from the accreditation process. Not Accredited is an appealable accreditation decision.

Requests for Revision to the *Official Accreditation Decision Report*

The organization has 30 days from receipt of its *Official Accreditation Decision Report* to request, in writing, a revision of any portion of the report related to survey findings or follow-up activity.

Appealing Not Accredited or Preliminarily Nonaccredited Decisions

The organization has 20 days from receipt of its *Official Accreditation Decision Report* to notify the Joint Commission, in writing, of its intent to appeal a decision to deny accreditation. An organization that has received written notice from the Joint Commission of being preliminarily denied accreditation or provisional accreditation has 20 days to make a written request for a hearing.

Award Display and Use

The Joint Commission provides each accredited organization with a certificate of accreditation. There is no charge for the initial certificate. Additional certificates may be purchased. Such requests should be sent to the Certificate Coordinator, Division of Accreditation Operations at the Joint Commission.

The certificate and all copies remain the Joint Commission's property. They must be returned if

- the organization is issued a new certificate reflecting a name change; or
- the organization's accreditation status is changed, withdrawn, or denied, for any reason.

An organization accredited by the Joint Commission must be accurate in describing to the public the nature and meaning of its accreditation and its award.* On request, the Joint Commission's Department of Communications will supply an organization receiving accreditation with appropriate guidelines for characterizing the accreditation award. Guidelines also cover accreditation with commendation awards.

An organization may not engage in any false or misleading advertising of the accreditation award. Any such advertising may be grounds to deny accreditation. For example, an organization may not represent its accreditation as being awarded by any of the Joint Commission's corporate members. These include the American College of Physicians, the American College of Surgeons, the American Dental Association, the American Hospital Association, and the American Medical Association. The Joint Commission has permission to reprint the seals of its corporate members on the certificates of accreditation. However, these seals must not be reproduced or displayed separately from the certificate.

Any organization that materially misleads the public about any matter relating to its accreditation must undertake corrective advertising of a degree acceptable to the Joint Commission in the same medium in which the misrepresentation occurred. If an organization fails to undertake the required corrective advertising following the communication of false or misleading advertising about its accreditation status, the organization may be subject to loss of accreditation.

The Joint Commission's logo is a registered trademark. An accredited organization may use the logo if it follows these guidelines:

- The logo must remain in the same proportional relationship as provided and should not be displayed any larger than an organization's own logo.
- The logo's format cannot be changed, the name may not be separated from the symbol, and they must be printed in the same color.
- Graphic devices such as seals, other words, or slogans cannot be added to the logo except for the words "Accredited by."

---

* See Requirement 10 on page 44 in the Accreditation Participation Requirements chapter.

These guidelines apply for logo use on all print materials and promotional items, such as coffee mugs, T-shirts, and note pads. Contact the Department of Communications at the Joint Commission at 630/792-5631 for questions about using the Joint Commission logo.

Before the Next Survey

This section provides information relevant to organizations between Joint Commission surveys. Material includes the duration of an accreditation award; the process for continuing accreditation; how to notify the Joint Commission in the event of organizational changes including mergers, consolidations, and acquisitions; and unscheduled and unannounced surveys.

Duration of Accreditation Award

An accreditation award is valid for three years, unless revoked for cause or as otherwise outlined in this chapter. Accreditation is effective on the first day after the Joint Commission completes the organization's survey. Organizations may request a full accreditation survey more frequently than once every three years. The Joint Commission will, at its discretion and in accordance with its mission, determine whether to honor the request. Such requests should be sent to the organization's accreditation service specialist.

Resolving Type I Recommendations. The Joint Commission requires an organization receiving a type I recommendation to achieve substantial or significant compliance with the relevant standard(s) within a specific time frame. Failure to do so can result in a conditional accreditation or not accredited decision.

The Joint Commission monitors an organization accredited with type I recommendations for their successful resolution. Monitoring and the time frame for demonstrating improvements depend on the nature of the type I recommendations. The potential impact on individual care is of particular concern. For many type I recommendations, the Joint Commission requires an organization to submit a written progress report. Other type I recommendations require an on-site survey known as a focused survey. The number of surveyors and the length of the focused survey may depend on the number and nature of the type I recommendations.

During a focused survey, surveyors may need to address standards other than those cited with a type I recommendation(s) to fully address compliance with the cited standards. Also, organizations are responsible for meeting the requirements of the most current standards—that is, the standards in effect at the time of the focused survey, which may be different from the standards that were in effect at the time the type I recommendation(s) was assigned.

Continuous Compliance. The Joint Commission expects an accredited organization to be in continuous compliance with all applicable standards. It may ask an organization to supply, in writing, information about standards compliance. Or it may survey an organization at any time, with or without notice. The Joint Commission may perform such surveys in response to complaints, media coverage, or other information-raising questions about standards compliance or the adequacy of individual health and safety protections (see "Unscheduled and Unannounced Surveys" on page 37). The Joint Commission might also conduct a survey if an organization fails to respond to a request for more information.

An organization's failure to permit a survey can be viewed by the Joint Commission as grounds to deny accreditation or as withdrawal by the organization from the accreditation process.*

* See Requirement 3 on page 40 in the Accreditation Participation Requirements chapter.

Continuing Accreditation

The Joint Commission does not automatically renew an organization's accreditation. An organization seeking to continue its accreditation must apply for accreditation, undergo a full accreditation survey, and be found in compliance with the standards.

Accreditation Renewal Process. The Joint Commission sends an organization an Application for Survey before the organization's triennial accreditation due date. The organization is responsible for completing and returning the Application for Survey to the Joint Commission.

The Joint Commission schedules a survey to determine an organization's eligibility to renew its accreditation award. This triennial survey occurs close to the end of the three-year accreditation cycle. Generally, the Joint Commission conducts a triennial survey in the time period between 45 days before the organization's three-year survey due date and 45 days after the due date. The Joint Commission notifies the organization of the survey date at least four weeks before the survey.

Accreditation Status During Triennial Survey. An organization's previous accreditation status remains in effect until a decision is made either to accredit or to preliminarily nonaccredit the organization.

Notification of Changes Made Between Surveys

Accreditation is neither automatically transferred nor continued if significant changes occur within the organization. Such changes may necessitate an extension of accreditation survey of the organization if the organization has

- instituted a new service or program for which the Joint Commission has standards;
- changed ownership and there are a significant number of changes in the management and clinical staff or operating policies and procedures;
- offered at least 25% of its services at a new location or in a significantly altered physical plant;
- expanded its capacity to provide services by 25% or more as measured by beds, individual visits, pieces of equipment, or other relevant measures;
- provided a more intensive level of service (for example, from outpatient alcohol and drug use to residential alcohol and drug use); or
- merged with, consolidated with, or acquired an unaccredited site, service, or program for which there are applicable Joint Commission standards.

An extension of accreditation survey may also occur when

- the Joint Commission grants an organization's request to continue its current accreditation beyond the conclusion of the three-year cycle;* or
- an organization has merged, consolidated, or acquired an accredited organization whose accreditation expiration date is within three months of the merger, consolidation, or acquisition, while its own accreditation expiration date is at least nine months away.

When any of these changes occur, the organization must notify the Joint Commission in writing not more than 30 days after such change is made. When an organization offers at least 25% of its services at a new location or in a significantly altered physical plant, the organization must also fill out and submit to the Joint Commission Part 2: Basic Building Information of the Statement of Conditions™. Failure to provide timely notification to the Joint Commission of these changes may result in the loss of accreditation.

An extension of accreditation survey is conducted at an accredited organization or at a site that is owned and operated by or that is publicly represented as being part of an accredited organization if the accredited organization's current accreditation is not due to expire for at least nine months and when at least one of the conditions above is met. The results of an extension of accreditation survey may affect the organization's accreditation status.

---

* Such requests are granted only for unusual and compelling reasons.

Mergers, Consolidations, and Acquisitions. In the case of a merger, consolidation, or acquisition, the Joint Commission may decide that the organization responsible for services must be resurveyed or initially surveyed. Barring exceptional circumstances, the Joint Commission continues the accreditation of the organization undergoing the kind of changes described above until it determines whether an extension of accreditation survey is necessary.

Annual Update Process

Beginning in 1998, all accredited health care organizations will be contacted by the Joint Commission on or around their triennial due date. Organizations will be contacted and asked to verify or correct key demographics maintained about their organization, including the selection of a performance measurement system and indicators as part of the ORYX Initiative. Once this demographic information is updated and verified, a certification form detailing the update will be sent to the health care organization. The organization will then be asked to verify and certify the information is correct and return it to the Joint Commission.

Unscheduled and Unannounced Surveys

The Joint Commission may perform either an unscheduled or unannounced survey when it becomes aware of potentially serious care or safety issues in an accredited organization.* Either type of survey can take place at *any* point in an organization's three-year accreditation cycle. The Joint Commission usually provides the organization with 24 to 48 hours advance notice of an *unscheduled survey*.

No advance notice is provided for *unannounced surveys*. Reasons for unannounced surveys include occurrence of any event or series of events in an accredited organization that creates significant

- concern that there may be a continuing threat to the safety or care of individuals;
- concern that there may be continuing serious and/or multiple significant standards compliance deficiency(ies); or
- suspicion that the organization is not or has not been in compliance with the Joint Commission's falsification policy.

Such a survey can either include all the organization's services or only those areas where a serious concern may exist.

Results of any unannounced or unscheduled surveys may generate appropriate follow-up activities and can affect an organization's current accreditation status. The Joint Commission may deny accreditation or conclude that the organization has withdrawn from the accreditation process if the organization does not let the Joint Commission conduct unscheduled or unannounced surveys.

Random Unannounced Surveys

The Joint Commission also conducts midcycle, unannounced surveys on a 5% random sample of accredited organizations. The survey is generally conducted 18 months following the accreditation date (that is, the date after the last day of the survey) plus or minus 30 days. An organization will receive a 24- to 48-hour notice of the random, unannounced survey. One surveyor conducts each such survey for one day.

The surveyor primarily assesses the five performance areas identified by the Joint Commission as the most troublesome in the previous year's aggregate survey data for the program to be surveyed and any additional performance areas as specified by the Accreditation Committee. These performance areas may change annually based on the previous year's data. Contact organization accreditation services for a current list of performance areas.

---

* See Requirement 3 on page 40 in the Accreditation Participation Requirements chapter.

Accreditation Participation Requirements

This chapter includes specific requirements for accreditation participation in the accreditation process and for maintenance of an accreditation award. The requirements in this chapter differ from survey eligibility criteria in that the accreditation process may be initiated even when all accreditation participation requirements have not yet been met. Requirements 1 through 3 and Requirements 7 through 10 are existing accreditation policies within the Accreditation Cycle chapter (see pages 5 through 38) and are currently effective for accreditation purposes. Therefore, organizations must be in current compliance with each of these requirements. Each requirement is cross-referenced to the applicable section of the Accreditation Cycle chapter. By contrast, Requirements 4, 5, and 6 are new and will be implemented incrementally over the next few years. Requirements 4 and 5 become effective for accreditation purposes on March 1, 1999; Requirement 6 becomes effective on January 1, 2000.

For a behavioral health care organization seeking accreditation for the first time, compliance with the accreditation participation requirements is assessed during the initial survey. For the accredited behavioral health care organization, compliance with these requirements is assessed throughout the accreditation cycle through on-site surveys, written progress reports, periodic updates of behavioral health care-specific data and information, and ad hoc communications. Starting March 1, 1999, when a behavioral health care organization that provides any 24-hour care does not fully comply with an accreditation participation requirement, the behavioral health care organization will usually be assigned a *special type I recommendation.* However, refusal to permit performance of an unscheduled or unannounced survey (Requirement 3) or falsification of information (Requirement 9), will immediately lead to preliminary nonaccreditation. Special type I recommendations can impact the accreditation decision, overall performance score, and follow-up requirements, as determined by established accreditation decision rules. Failure to resolve a special type I recommendation can ultimately lead to loss of accreditation.

Application for Survey

Requirement 1 The behavioral health care organization provides the Joint Commission with all official records and reports of public or publicly recognized licensing (for example, a state license), examining, reviewing, or planning bodies.*

Requirement 2 The behavioral health care organization immediately reports any changes in the information provided in the Application for Survey.†

A behavioral health care organization that experiences a significant change in ownership or control, location, capacity, or the categories of services offered must notify the Joint Commission in writing not more than 30 days after such changes. The Joint Commission may decide that the behavioral health care organization must be resurveyed when a significant merger or consolidation has taken place. The Joint Commission continues the behavioral health care organization's accreditation until it determines whether a resurvey is necessary. Failure to provide timely notification to the Joint Commission of ownership, merger or consolidation, and service changes may result in interruption or loss of accreditation. When requested, the behavioral health care organization is required to provide the Joint Commission with all official records and reports of public or publicly recognized licensing, examining, reviewing, or planning bodies.

Compliance with Requirement 1 ❑ Yes
❑ No

Compliance with Requirement 2 ❑ Yes
❑ No

Acceptance of Survey

Requirement 3 A behavioral health care organization permits the performance of an unscheduled or unannounced survey‡ at the discretion of the Joint Commission.

The Joint Commission may perform either an unscheduled or unannounced survey when it becomes aware of potentially serious patient care or safety issues in a behavioral health care organization. Either type of survey can take place at any point in a behavioral health care organization's three-year accreditation cycle. An unscheduled or unannounced survey can either include all of the behavioral health care organization's services or address only those areas where a serious concern may exist. In addition, the Joint Commission conducts unannounced surveys on a random sample of accredited behavioral health care organizations at the approximate midpoint of their three-year accreditation cycles. A behavioral health care organization's failure to permit an unscheduled or unannounced survey is grounds for withdrawal of accreditation.

Compliance with Requirement 3 ❑ Yes
❑ No

---

* See also page 23 in the Accreditation Cycle chapter.

† See also page 24 in the Accreditation Cycle chapter.

‡ See also page 37 in the Accreditation Cycle chapter. An explanation of the difference between an unscheduled and un-announced survey can be found on these pages. In addition, see the last paragraph of "Continuous Compliance" on page 35.

Performance Measurement

Requirement 4 The behavioral health care organization that provides any 24-hour care participates in a listed performance measurement system that has been found to be acceptable for use in the accreditation process.

Each of these behavioral health care organizations must select at least one performance measurement system that is listed by the Joint Commission as acceptable for use in the accreditation process. Each accredited behavioral health care organization must notify the Joint Commission of its initial selection(s) prior to March 1, 1999. A behavioral health care organization applying for initial survey must notify the Joint Commission of its selection(s) no later than the last day of the initial survey. Each behavioral health care organization must notify the Joint Commission of any changes in its relationship with the selected performance measurement system(s) or the selection of a new or additional performance measurement system used to meet performance measurement reporting requirements.

Note: *Accredited behavioral health care organizations that do not provide any 24-hour care must participate in a request for indicators (RFI) project conducted by the Joint Commission to identify performance measures currently being used to meet performance improvement standards. The responses will be used to create a template of measures from which the organizations will select measures. They must also select at least two measures from the template and inform the Joint Commission of its selection by June 30, 1999, and begin collecting data for selected measures from third quarter 1999 by July 1, 1999. Organizations will be expected to share data, and analyze conclusions and actions with surveyors during regular, on-site surveys beginning January 1, 2000.*

Compliance with Requirement 4 ❑ Yes
❑ No

Requirement 5 The behavioral health care organization that provides any 24-hour care selects and uses indicators from at least one listed performance measurement system.

The behavioral health care organization identifies clinical, client perception of care, or health status indicators that meet Joint Commission requirements for the number of indicators and percentage of individual population covered. The number of indicators and percentage of individual population monitored will increase over time. The behavioral health care organization submits data for its indicators to the performance measurement system(s) at least quarterly, and such submissions identify monthly data points. Each accredited behavioral health care organization must notify the Joint Commission of its initial indicator selections prior to March 1, 1999. A behavioral health care organization applying for initial survey must notify the Joint Commission of its indicator selection(s) no later than the last day of the initial survey. Each behavioral health care organization must also notify the Joint Commission of any subsequent additions or changes to its indicator selections. An individual indicator must be used for at least four consecutive quarters. For purposes of reporting to the Joint Commission, a behavioral health care organization will be expected to

- continue to use an indicator if the indicator data suggest an unstable pattern of performance or otherwise identify an opportunity for improvement; or
- change to a new indicator if the indicator data reflect continuing stable and satisfactory performance.

Note: *Between the years 1999 and 2002, the minimum number of required measures and percentage of individual population monitored by the selected measures will increase according to the following schedule:*

Year	Minimum Number of Selected Measures	Maximum Number of Selected Measures	Minimum Percentage of Individual Population Monitored
1999	2	5	20%
2000	4	8	25%
2001	6	10	30%
2002	8	12	35%

Note: *Accredited behavioral health care organizations that do not provide any 24-hour care must participate in a request for indicators (RFI) project conducted by the Joint Commission to identify performance measures currently being used to meet performance improvement standards. The responses will be used to create a template of measures from which the organizations will select measures. They must also select at least two measures from the template and inform the Joint Commission of its selection by June 30, 1999, and begin collecting data for selected measures from third quarter 1999 by July 1, 1999. Organizations will be expected to share data, and analyze conclusions and actions with surveyors during regular, on-site surveys beginning January 1, 2000.*

Compliance with Requirement 5
- ❑ Yes
- ❑ No

Requirement 6 The behavioral health care organization that provides any 24-hour care ensures that aggregate data for the selected indicators are submitted to the Joint Commission at least quarterly.

Behavioral health care-specific aggregate data, which include monthly data points, must be submitted quarterly to the Joint Commission for use in the accreditation process. Findings based on the Joint Commission's analysis of the data may lead to subsequent intracycle monitoring activities. The quarterly data submissions must begin no later than March 31, 2000. The Joint Commission will define the type and format of performance measurement data to be submitted in a fashion consistent with nationally-recognized standards.

The submission of behavioral health care-specific data will be performed by the performance measurement system(s) and will include comparative data for other behavioral health care organizations that have selected these same performance measures.

Note: *Accredited behavioral health care organizations that do not provide any 24-hour care must participate in a request for indicators (RFI) project conducted by the Joint Commission to identify performance measures currently being used to meet performance improvement standards. The responses will be used to create a template of measures from which the organizations will select measures. They must also select at least two measures from the template and inform the Joint Commission of its selection by June 30, 1999.*

Compliance with Requirement 6
- ❑ Yes
- ❑ Data have not been submitted for one of four consecutive quarters
- ❑ Data have not been submitted for more than one of four consecutive quarters

Public Information Interviews

Requirement 7 The behavioral health care organization provides notice of an upcoming full accreditation survey and of the opportunity for a public information interview.*

A behavioral health care organization must provide an opportunity for the public to participate in a public information interview during a full survey. The public includes

- individuals and their families;
- personal advocates;
- members of the community for whom services are provided; and
- behavioral health care organization personnel.

To comply with the 30-day policy for notifying the public about the upcoming survey, the behavioral health care organization is responsible for making the public information interview process widely known and effective as a source of compliance information in the accreditation process. The Joint Commission requires a behavioral health care organization scheduled for a full survey to post announcements of the survey date and of the opportunity for a public information interview. To maximize participation, postings must be made throughout the behavioral health care organization in the form provided by the Joint Commission. Behavioral health care organizations should post notices in public eating areas, on bulletin boards near major entrances, and in treatment or residential areas. In addition, if all staff members are not likely to see such postings, the behavioral health care organization must provide each staff member with a written announcement of the survey.

The behavioral health care organization must also provide potential public information interview participants with sufficient advance notice. The Joint Commission requires behavioral health care organizations to post public notices at least 30 days before the scheduled survey date. Notices must remain posted until the survey is completed.

The behavioral health care organization should also promptly initiate community advertisement or other communications as soon as it receives notice of the survey date. Appropriate steps to take in notifying the community of the opportunity for public information interviews include

- informing organized patient advocacy groups that have substantively communicated with the behavioral health care organization in the previous 12 months;
- reaching other members of the community, for example through a classified advertisement in a local newspaper or newsletter; and
- informing individuals who inquire about the survey of the survey date(s) and opportunity to participate.

Compliance with Requirement 7 ❑ Yes
❑ No

Requirement 8 The behavioral health care organization notifies the Joint Commission of any requests for a public information interview.†

The behavioral health care organization must promptly forward to the Joint Commission all written requests to participate in a public information interview. Behavioral health care organizations receiving an oral request should instruct the individual(s) to make the request in writing and mail it to the Joint Commission. The behavioral health care organization should provide the individual(s) needing assistance in doing this with the necessary support. The behavioral health care organization

---

* See also pages 26 through 28 in the Accreditation Cycle chapter.

† See also pages 27–28 in the Accreditation Cycle chapter.

is responsible for notifying the interviewee(s) of the exact date, time, and place of the public information interview.

Compliance with Requirement 8 ❑ Yes
❑ No

Misrepresentation of Information

Requirement 9 The behavioral health care organization does not misrepresent information in the accreditation process.*

Information provided by the behavioral health care organization and used by the Joint Commission for the accreditation process must be accurate and truthful. Such information may

- be provided orally;
- be obtained through direct observation by Joint Commission surveyors;
- be derived from documents supplied by the behavioral health care organization to the Joint Commission; and
- involve data submitted electronically by the behavioral health care organization to the Joint Commission.

The Joint Commission requires each behavioral health care organization seeking accreditation to engage in the accreditation process in good faith. Any behavioral health care organization that fails to participate in good faith by falsifying information presented in the accreditation process may have its accreditation denied or removed by the Joint Commission.

For the purpose of this requirement, falsification is defined as the fabrication, in whole or in part, of any information provided by an applicant or accredited behavioral health care organization to the Joint Commission. This includes any redrafting, reformatting, or content deletion of documents. However, the behavioral health care organization may submit additional material that summarizes or otherwise explains the original information submitted to the Joint Commission. These additional materials must be properly identified, dated, and accompanied by the original documents.

Compliance with Requirement 9 ❑ Yes
❑ No

Requirement 10 The behavioral health care organization does not publicly misrepresent its accreditation status or the scope of facilities and services to which the accreditation applies.†

Behavioral health care organizations accredited by the Joint Commission must be accurate when describing to the public the nature and meaning of their accreditation. On request, the Joint Commission's Department of Communications will provide accredited behavioral health care organizations with appropriate guidelines for characterizing the accreditation award. These guidelines also cover accreditation with commendation awards. A behavioral health care organization may not engage in any false or misleading advertising with respect to the accreditation award. Any such advertising may be grounds for denying or revoking accreditation.

Compliance with Requirement 10 ❑ Yes
❑ No

---

* See also page 13 in the Accreditation Cycle chapter.

† See also page 34 in the Accreditation Cycle chapter.

Rights, Responsibilities, and Ethics

Overview

The **goal** of the rights, responsibilities, and ethics function is to improve care, services, and outcomes by recognizing and respecting each individual, in accordance with fundamental human, civil, constitutional, and statutory rights.

Care and services are provided in such a way as to respect and foster in individuals served a sense of dignity, autonomy, positive self-regard, civil rights, and involvement in the provision of their own care and services. This involvement takes into account the individuals' strengths, weaknesses, and resources; the relevant demands of their environments; and the requirements and expectations of the service providers and those they serve.

Standards

A list of all standards for this function appears below, presented without footnotes or other explanatory text. If you have any questions about a term used here, please refer to the standard as it appears in the next section of this chapter—Standards and Intent Statements.

RI.1 Using a framework that reflects the interdependence of care and service delivery and organizational ethical issues, the organization addresses the rights of individuals served and ethical issues in the delivery of care and services.

RI.1.1 The organization respects the rights of individuals served to receive care or services within its capability, mission, and applicable law and regulation.

RI.1.2 Individuals served are involved in all aspects of care and service, in accordance with approved policies and as appropriate to the setting or service.

RI.1.2.1 Individuals served receive adequate information about the clinical staff responsible for their care.

RI.1.2.2 Informed consent is obtained from each individual served.

RI.1.2.3 The organization involves family members, when appropriate, in facilitating care decisions.

RI.1.2.4 Individuals involved in investigational studies and clinical trials participate in care decisions throughout the care process.

RI.1.2.5 Individuals served are involved in resolving conflicts in care decisions.

RI.1.2.6 Individuals who want pastoral services have access to them, as appropriate to the treatment setting or service.

RI.1.3 A framework for decision making in the care of dying individuals is reflected in the planning and delivery of care and services, as appropriate to the setting or service.

RI.1.4 The organization respects the need for confidentiality of information concerning each individual served and the individual's family.

RI.1.5 The organization respects the need for privacy and security of each individual served and the individual's family.

RI.1.6 The organization respects the need for communication of each individual served and, when appropriate, the individual's family.

RI.1.6.1 If therapeutic indications necessitate restrictions on visitors, mail, telephone calls, or other forms of communication, those restrictions are evaluated for their therapeutic effectiveness.

RI.1.6.1.1 All such restrictions are fully explained and determined with the participation of the individual served and, when appropriate, the individual's family.

RI.1.6.2 All individuals are informed of their rights in a language they understand.

RI.1.6.3 When people who speak various languages make substantial use of the organization, personnel who speak their language(s) are available.

RI.1.6.4 As appropriate, personnel are available who can effectively communicate with people who have hearing and speech impairments.

RI.1.7 The organization respects the need for resolving complaints of each individual served and the individual's family.

RI.1.8 All individuals served receive a written statement of their rights.

RI.2 The rights of individuals are protected and respected during research, experimentation, or clinical trials involving human subjects.

RI.2.1 Before requesting their consent for participation, all individuals asked to participate in a research project are given full explanations of

RI.2.1.1 the benefits to be expected;

RI.2.1.2 the potential discomforts and risks;

RI.2.1.3 alternative services that might benefit them;

RI.2.1.4 the procedures to be followed, especially those that are experimental in nature; and

RI.2.1.5 their right to refuse to participate in any research project without compromising their access to the organization's services.

RI.2.2 Documentation of consent includes all the information specified in RI.2.1.1 through RI.2.1.5, the name of the staff member who supplied the information, with the staff member's signature and date, and addresses the participant's right to privacy, confidentiality, and safety.

RI.2.3 When research procedures are completed, the principal investigator attempts to alleviate, to the extent possible, any confusion, misinformation, stress, physical discomfort, or other harmful consequences that participants may have experienced as a result of research procedures.

RI.3 Policies and procedures govern vocational rehabilitation services in which individuals served work for the service provider as part of their treatment.

RI.4 Individuals served can obtain a personal advocate when appropriate.

RI.5 Clinical staff help individuals served, their families, and the court determine the need for protective services.

RI.6 Individuals served, their families, and the courts are assisted in determining the need for guardianship through an independent assessment that ensures the individual served is the primary beneficiary.

RI.7 Use of special treatment procedures is consistent with the rights of individuals served and organization policies governing their use.

RI.8 The organization has a code of ethical behavior.

RI.8.1 The code addresses ethical issues in the provision of care and services to individuals served.

RI.8.2 The code addresses marketing, admission, and billing practices.

RI.8.3 The code addresses organization and staff relationships to other health care providers, educational institutions, and payers.

RI.8.4 The code addresses the protection of the integrity of clinical decision making regardless of how the organization compensates, or shares financial risk with, its leaders, managers, clinical staff, and licensed independent practitioners.

Standards and Intent Statements

Rights and Responsibilities

Standard

RI.1 Using a framework that reflects the interdependence of care and service delivery and organizational ethical issues, the organization addresses the rights of individuals served and ethical issues in the delivery of care and services.

Intent of RI.1

Simply listing the rights of individuals served cannot ensure those rights will be respected. This standard focuses on the organization's efforts to reflect concern and respect for the rights of individuals served during all its interactions with those individuals, on increasing staff awareness of the ethical issues surrounding the provision of care and services, on the organization's policies governing such issues, and on the methods available to support ethical decision making.

The organization supports the following rights of individuals served:

- The right to reasonable access to care, regardless of race, religion, gender, sexual orientation, ethnicity, age, or disability;
- The right to personal dignity;
- The right to care that is considerate and respects the personal value and belief systems of individuals served;
- The right to be informed of the organization's rules and regulations concerning the conduct of the individuals served;
- The right to informed participation in decisions regarding care and services;
- The right to participate in treatment planning including children as appropriate to their age, maturity, and clinical condition,* and the right of the family[†] of individuals served to participate in such planning;
- The right to individualized treatment, including:
  - adequate and humane services regardless of the source(s) of financial support,
  - provision of services within the least restrictive environment possible,
  - an individualized treatment or program plan,
  - periodic review of the treatment or program plan, and
  - an adequate number of competent, qualified, and experienced professional clinical staff to supervise and carry out the treatment or program plan;
- The right to participate in the consideration of ethical issues that arise in the provision of care and services, including:
  - resolving conflict,
  - withholding resuscitative services,
  - forgoing or withdrawing life-sustaining treatment, and

---

* Depending on state rules and regulations

[†] **family** The person(s) who plays a significant role in the member's life, which may include an individual(s) not legally related to the member. This person(s) is often referred to as a surrogate decision maker, if authorized to make care decisions for a member who loses decision-making capacity.

  - participating in investigational studies or clinical trials;
- The right to personal privacy and confidentiality of information;
- The right to designate a surrogate decision maker* if the individual served is incapable of understanding a proposed treatment or procedure or is unable to communicate his or her wishes regarding care; and
- The right of the individual served and the individual's family to be informed of their rights in a language that they understand.

Access

Standard

RI.1.1 The organization respects the rights of individuals served to receive care or services within its capability, mission, and applicable law and regulation.

Intent of RI.1.1

In response to the request and needs of individuals it can serve, the organization provides care and services that are within its capacity, its stated mission and philosophy, and applicable law and regulation. The organization uses a defined referral process to help individuals locate needed services the organization cannot provide.

When requested or needed care is beyond the organization's capability or is in conflict with its mission or philosophy, the individual may be transferred to another facility when clinically permissible. The reasons for any proposed transfer are communicated and discussed with the individual and, as appropriate, the individual's family. When limits to the lengths of available treatment are dictated by reimbursement issues, the individual is informed as part of the entry process that an appropriate transfer may be made. That transfer is made only after the individual has received complete information and an explanation concerning the needs for, and alternatives to, such a transfer. The transfer must be acceptable to the receiving organization.

Care

Standard

RI.1.2 Individuals served are involved in all aspects of care† and service, in accordance with approved policies and as appropriate to the setting or service.

Intent of RI.1.2

The organization defines how individuals will be involved in all aspects of their care. The mechanisms for involvement are developed in consultation with clinical and other appropriate staff and approved by appropriate leaders. This process ensures broad input, cross-organizational communication, and alignment with the organization's mission and resources.

---

* **surrogate decision maker** Someone appointed to act on behalf of another. Surrogates make decisions only when an individual is without capacity or has given permission to involve others, such as a legal guardian.

† "Care" includes care, treatment, services, rehabilitation, habilitation, or other programs instituted for the individual served.

Standard

RI.1.2.1 Individuals served receive adequate information about the clinical staff responsible for their care.

Intent of RI.1.2.1

The organization gives individuals served enough information about staff members who are responsible for the delivery of their care and services to meet their needs. Information provided to each individual includes:

- the identity of the physician, practitioner, or provider who has primary responsibility for the care and services provided;
- the identity and professional status of persons responsible for authorizing and performing procedures or treatments;
- notice of, and reasons for, any proposed change in the clinical staff responsible for the individual's care; and
- an explanation of any professional relationships among people who are treating the individual, and to any other health care or educational institutions involved in the individual's care.

Standard

RI.1.2.2 Informed consent is obtained from each individual served.

Intent of RI.1.2.2

Informed consent is a process. Individuals are given a clear, concise explanation of

- their condition;
- proposed interventions, treatment, or medications;
- the potential benefits, risks, and side effects of proposed interventions, treatment, or medications;
- problems related to recovery;
- the likelihood of success;
- any significant alternative medications, treatments, or interventions; and
- the individual's right, to the extent permitted by law, to refuse medications, treatments, or interventions.

Standard

RI.1.2.3 The organization involves family members, when appropriate, in facilitating care decisions.

Intent of RI.1.2.3

When appropriate, the organization may involve family members in facilitating care decisions when circumstances require that people other than, or in addition to, the individual served be involved in decisions about the individual's care. In the case of an unemancipated minor, the family or guardian is legally responsible for approval of care.

Standard

RI.1.2.4 Individuals involved in investigational studies and clinical trials participate in care decisions throughout the care process.

Intent of RI.1.2.4

Individuals served have the right to be informed of any experimental, research, or educational activities involved in their treatment. Individuals served also have the right to refuse to participate, or withdraw consent and discontinue participation, in any such activity.

Standard

RI.1.2.5 Individuals served are involved in resolving conflicts in care decisions.

Intent of RI.1.2.5

The organization has defined a process for reviewing and assessing the needs, requests, and complaints about care communicated by individuals served and families. All populations served have access to such a process. In addition, individuals served have the right to request the opinion of a consultant at their expense or to request an in-house review of the individual treatment plan, as outlined in organization procedures.

The conflict-resolution process is developed by clinical and other staff and is appropriately approved. The organization also defines the final authority for addressing admission, treatment, and discharge issues. When individuals refuse treatment, they are given full information about the organization's responsibility to seek appropriate legal alternatives or orders of involuntary treatment, or, in accordance with professional standards, to terminate the relationship between the individual served and the provider upon reasonable notice.

Standard

RI.1.2.6 Individuals who want pastoral services have access to them, as appropriate to the treatment setting or service.

Intent of RI.1.2.6

Each individual served has access to pastoral services provided directly by the organization or through a working relationship with local clergy. These services may include pastoral care, religious consultation, and education. When pastoral services are provided by the facility, written policies and procedures govern their operation.

Standard

RI.1.3 A framework for decision making in the care of dying individuals is reflected in the planning and delivery of care and services, as appropriate to the setting or service.

Intent of RI.1.3

The psychosocial, spiritual, and cultural values that affect the individual's response to care are considered in care planning and delivery. Individuals served are allowed to express spiritual beliefs and cultural practices that do not harm others or interfere with the planned course of care and services.

Sensitivity to needs and values of the individual served is especially important in care for the dying. Organization policies and procedures promote staff awareness of, and responsiveness to, these special needs. To ensure that care and services provided to the dying are responsive and respectful, the goals of care and services include

- fostering the individual's comfort and dignity;

- providing appropriate treatment for primary and secondary symptoms that respond to treatment, as desired by the individual or the individual's designated representative;
- effectively managing pain; and
- responding to the individual's and family's psychosocial, spiritual, and cultural concerns and values.

Support provided for the psychological, social, emotional, and spiritual needs of the individual and family demonstrates respect for the individual's values, belief system, and life philosophy.

Policies and procedures address formulating advance directives.* As required by law and regulation, individuals served are informed of their right to formulate advance directives. When appropriate, the organization determines the existence of an advance directive or the identity of a surrogate decision maker. These policies apply to all adult individuals served, not just those who are dying, and to individuals of other ages when appropriate. In accordance with written policies and procedures, any known advance directives are considered during the treatment-planning process. Particular attention to advance directives is necessary in developing pain treatment or pain management plans. The absence of advance directives, however, should not hamper access to care. For some adults, this discussion may not be appropriate when first "entering" the organization, but will be addressed later in the course of treatment. If the individual does not have an advance directive but wants to develop one, the organization at least offers the individual a referral source.

Policies and procedures address decisions to withhold resuscitative services and decisions to forgo or withdraw life-sustaining treatment. No single policy can anticipate every situation that may demand difficult decisions about withholding resuscitative services or forgoing or withdrawing life-sustaining treatment. However, organizations can develop a framework for decision making in these cases, which will help identify the organization's position on initiating resuscitative services as well as using and removing life-sustaining treatment.

Decision-making mechanisms for these situations offer guidance to health professionals. These mechanisms address the ethical and legal issues involved in withholding resuscitative services or forgoing or withdrawing life-sustaining treatment and decrease the uncertainty about the practices permitted by the organization. It is vital that these mechanisms be formally adopted and approved by appropriate leaders of the organization to ensure internal consistency and accountability for decisions made.

Mechanisms that guide decision making about resuscitative services and life-sustaining treatment will need to conform to applicable legal requirements. They will also provide for modification of such decisions as the individual progresses through the episode of care.

Decision making about care at the end of life involves individuals served and their families and reflects consideration of special issues related to care for the dying. Care that is responsive to the needs of the individuals served at the end of life requires considering special issues and needs connected to this important and highly personal time. Decision making in the care of individuals who are dying reflects the following priorities:

- Fostering the individual's comfort and dignity by addressing treatment of primary and secondary symptoms;
- Effectively managing pain; and
- Responding to the individual's and family's specific psychosocial, spiritual, and cultural needs and concerns.

---

* **advance directives** A legal document allowing a person to give directions about future medical care or to designate another person(s) to make medical decisions if he or she should lose decision-making capability. Advance directives may include living wills, durable powers of attorney, or similar documents portraying the preference of the individual served.

Respect

Standards

RI.1.4 The organization respects the need for confidentiality of information concerning each individual served and the individual's family.

RI.1.5 The organization respects the need for privacy and security of each individual served and the individual's family.

RI.1.6 The organization respects the need for communication of each individual served and, when appropriate, the individual's family.

RI.1.6.1 If therapeutic indications necessitate restrictions on visitors, mail, telephone calls, or other forms of communication, those restrictions are evaluated for their therapeutic effectiveness.

RI.1.6.1.1 All such restrictions are fully explained and determined with the participation of the individual served and, when appropriate, the individual's family.

RI.1.6.2 All individuals are informed of their rights in a language they understand.

RI.1.6.3 When people who speak various languages make substantial use of the organization, personnel who speak their language(s) are available.

RI.1.6.4 As appropriate, personnel are available who can effectively communicate* with people who have hearing and speech impairments.

RI.1.7 The organization respects the need for resolving complaints of each individual served and the individual's family.

RI.1.8 All individuals served receive a written statement of their rights.

Intent of RI.1.4 Through RI.1.8

In addition to the influence of cultural, psychosocial, and spiritual beliefs on the course of care, other issues concerning respect influence care, such as

- privacy and security within the constraints of the treatment plan;
- the individual's and family's right to initiate a complaint or grievance procedure and to have complaints reviewed and, when possible, resolved;
- effective communication in the language of the population group(s) served;
- the right to confidentiality of information;
- the right of visitation by family and significant others, unless clinically contraindicated;
- the right to send and receive mail without hindrance; and
- the right to conduct private telephone conversations.

Full information is given to the individual served on the current and future use of special observation and audiovisual techniques, such as one-way mirrors, tape recorders, television, movies, or photographs.

* **effective communication** Any form of communication (for example writing, speech) that leads to demonstrable understanding.

If therapeutic indications necessitate restrictions on visitors, telephone calls, or other communications, those restrictions are evaluated for therapeutic effectiveness by the clinically responsible staff. Such limitations are determined with the participation of the individual and the individual's family and are fully explained to them. Clinically responsible staff evaluate any restrictions for therapeutic effectiveness at least every three days or at intervals consistent with ongoing care review and the average length of stay in the organization.

All individuals served receive a written statement of their rights in a language they understand while they are receiving treatment within the organization. Individuals who are disoriented or in a state of anxiety at the time of admission are informed of their rights at an appropriate time during treatment. Statements of rights are available to individuals served throughout treatment.

Research, Experimentation, and Clinical Trials

Standard

RI.2 The rights of individuals are protected and respected during research, experimentation, or clinical trials involving human subjects.

Intent of RI.2

When an organization conducts research, experimentation, or clinical trials involving human subjects, it establishes policies and procedures governing these activities. A research review committee is established to review all projects in relation to

- the mission statement;
- other organization guidelines;
- the project's values;
- its relative risks and benefits to the subject(s); and
- the process for obtaining the subject's consent.

Investigators and others directly involved in conducting human subject research or obtaining consent adhere to professional standards concerning the conduct of such research. They comply with the regulations of the U.S. Department of Health and Human Services and applicable law and regulation concerning the protection of human rights.

Standards

RI.2.1 *Before requesting their consent for participation, all individuals asked to participate in a research project are given full explanations of*

RI.2.1.1 the benefits to be expected;

RI.2.1.2 the potential discomforts and risks;

RI.2.1.3 alternative services that might benefit them;

RI.2.1.4 the procedures to be followed, especially those that are experimental in nature; and

RI.2.1.5 their right to refuse to participate in any research project without compromising their access to the organization's services.

RI.2.2 *Documentation of consent includes all the information specified in RI.2.1.1 through RI.2.1.5, the name of the staff member who supplied the information, with the staff member's signature and date, and addresses the participant's right to privacy, confidentiality, and safety.*

Intent of RI.2.1 Through RI.2.2

An organization that conducts research, investigations, or clinical trials involving human subjects knows that its first responsibility is to the health and well-being of the individuals served. To protect and respect the rights of individuals served, the organization always

- reviews all research protocols in relation to the organization's mission statement, values, and other guidelines;
- weighs the relative risks and benefits to the subjects; and
- obtains the subject's consent.

Valid, written individual consent must be obtained before an individual participates in a research project. Informed consent becomes possible when a competent individual is given the information needed to make a rational decision about whether to participate. Whether competent or not, individuals served have the right to refuse to participate in any research project without compromising their access to organization services. RI.2.1.1 through RI.2.1.5 identify the minimum and critical categories of information needed to provide a foundation for written informed consent.

Because the decision of the individual served to participate in clinical trials or research needs to be based on the individual's competency and sound information, the following items are documented in the individual's record:

- The name of the person who provided the information; and
- The date the form was signed.

Standard

RI.2.3 When research procedures are completed, the principal investigator attempts to alleviate, to the extent possible, any confusion, misinformation, stress, physical discomfort, or other harmful consequences that participants may have experienced as a result of research procedures.

Intent of RI.2.3

Research is conducted in a manner that respects the rights and needs of individuals served, and every effort is made to minimize potential adverse effects of participation in research. The principal investigator assumes responsibility for timely post-research follow-up with participants.

Work Programs for Individuals Served

Standard

RI.3 Policies and procedures govern vocational rehabilitation services in which individuals served work for the service provider as part of their treatment.

Intent of RI.3

The organization's primary responsibility to the individuals served is to provide treatment services. Treatment must not be compromised by using individuals to perform work for the organization. However, developing individuals through vocational rehabilitation programs to improve their skills or develop new ones may be considered an important part of treatment in some organizations. Practicing work skills would be considered a good experience in seeking jobs. In such instances, work activities of the individuals served and the rationale for them are reflected in the treatment-planning process.

Additional Interventions

Standard

RI.4 Individuals served can obtain a personal advocate when appropriate.

Intent of RI.4

The organization's process for providing a personal advocate for individuals served is described in writing. The description defines the conditions under which a personal advocate is indicated and the role and responsibilities of the personal advocate. Staff and individuals served are informed of the process.

Standard

RI.5 Clinical staff help individuals served, their families, and the court determine the need for protective services.

Intent of RI.5

Clinical staff members clearly define in writing their role in assessing the need for protective services, making recommendations based on assessment findings, and providing protective services. When the organization does not provide protective services, the clinical staff helps determine the need for such services and establishes necessary referral channels.

Standard

RI.6 Individuals served, their families, and the courts are assisted in determining the need for guardianship through an independent assessment that ensures the individual served is the primary beneficiary.

Intent of RI.6

The organization holds the interests of the individuals served above all others in assessing the need for guardianship. Recommendations concerning the need for guardianship are based on a separate review process independent of considerations used in the planning and delivery of care and services.

Standard

RI.7 Use of special treatment procedures is consistent with the rights of individuals served and organization policies governing their use.

Intent of RI.7

Special treatment procedures are used only after less restrictive procedures have proven ineffective. These procedures are used in accordance with the organization's policies and applicable law and regulation protecting the rights of the individuals served.

Special treatment procedures include, but are not necessarily limited to,

- seclusion;
- restraint;

- electroconvulsive therapy and other forms of convulsive therapy;
- unusual medications and investigational and experimental drugs;
- maintenance-use drugs that have abuse potential (usually considered to be controlled substances and drugs which can be used as chemical restraints);
- drugs that are known to involve a substantial risk or are associated with adverse drug reactions; and
- research projects that involve inconvenience or risk to the individuals served.

All special treatment procedures require clinical justification. The clinical indications for using special treatment procedures outweigh the known contraindications. Psychiatric care of children or adolescents may include the use of medications for purposes or in doses that, while not specifically approved for children and adolescents by the Food and Drug Administration, are not considered unusual by clinicians.

Organization Ethics

Standards

RI.8 The organization has a code of ethical behavior.

RI.8.1 The code addresses ethical issues in the provision of care and services to individuals served.

RI.8.2 The code addresses marketing, admission, and billing practices.

RI.8.3 The code addresses organization and staff relationships to other health care providers, educational institutions, and payers.

Intent of RI.8 Through RI.8.3

A health care organization has an ethical responsibility to the individuals and community it serves. To fulfill this responsibility, ethical care practices and ethical business practices must go hand in hand. The organization depends on its mission statement, strategic plan, and other such guiding documents to provide a consistent, ethical framework for its business operations.

In particular, the organization's code of ethical behavior ensures marketing and admission practices are conducted in an ethical manner. Individuals are billed for only those services received, which are summarized in an itemized list. Individuals receive full information about the organization's source of reimbursement for their care. Individuals are informed as soon as possible about any limitations placed on duration of services.

Potential conflicts of interest can arise in the most subtle of circumstances, as well as very obvious ones. Leaders need to be alert to the entire range of possibilities, review relationships with other entities carefully, and ensure that the organization's mission to the individuals and community it serves is not harmed by any contractual relationship.

Standard

RI.8.4 The code addresses the protection of the integrity of clinical decision making regardless of how the organization compensates, or shares financial risk with, its leaders, managers, clinical staff, and licensed independent practitioners.

Intent of RI.8.4

To avoid compromising the quality of care, clinical decisions including tests, treatments, and other interventions, are based on individuals' identified care needs. The organization's code of ethical business and professional behavior specifies that the organization implements policies and procedures that address this issue. Policies and procedures and information about the relationship between the use of services and financial incentives are available on request to all individuals served, the public, clinical staff, licensed independent practitioners, and organization personnel.

Assessment

Overview

The **goal** of the assessment function is to determine appropriate care through continuous assessment of each individual's needs. Qualified staff assess* individuals' care† needs throughout their contact with the organization. Identifying and delivering appropriate care depends on three processes:

1. *Collecting data.* Data‡ are collected about individuals' biopsychosocial needs and functioning, as appropriate to the setting and circumstances.
2. *Analyzing data.* Data are analyzed to produce information§ about individuals' needs for care and services and to identify the need for additional data.
3. *Making care decisions.* Approaches to meeting individuals' care needs are selected based on information generated through assessment.

An initial screening process may be completed at admission and contributes to the overall assessment process. Each individual might be screened for biopsychosocial needs and functioning that may require additional assessments, referrals, exceptional supervision, or intervention. The results of this screening would then serve as the basis for the initial treatment plan. The depth of the assessment depends on a number of factors, including individual needs, program goals, the anticipated length of stay, transfer, discharge, and aftercare needs.

---

* **assessment** The systematic collection and review of individual-specific data necessary to determine individual care needs.

† "Care" encompasses the care, treatment, services, rehabilitation, habilitation, or another program instituted for the individual served by the organization.

‡ **data** Uninterpreted sets of data that can assist in decision making.

§ **information** Interpreted sets of data that can assist in decision making.

Standards

A list of all standards for this function appears below, presented without footnotes or other explanatory text. If you have any questions about a term used here, please refer to the standard as it appears in the next section of this chapter—Standards and Intent Statements.

PE.1 Each individual's physical and psychological status and social functioning are assessed.

PE.1.1 An initial screening and/or assessment of each individual's physical, psychological, and social status is conducted to determine the need for care, the type of care to be provided, and the need for any further assessment.

PE.1.2 The organization has an assessment or screening procedure for the early detection of mental illness that is life threatening, indicates severe personality disorganization or deterioration, or may seriously affect the treatment or rehabilitation process.

PE.1.3 The need for assessing each individual's nutritional status is determined.

PE.1.4 The need for assessing the full range of each individual's functional status is determined.

PE.1.4.1 An assessment of physical functioning is performed for each individual referred for physical rehabilitation services.

PE.1.5 An emotional and behavioral assessment of each individual is completed and entered in the clinical record. The assessment includes at least a history of emotional, behavioral, and substance-abuse problems, their co-occurrence or treatment, including

PE.1.5.1 use of alcohol and other drugs by the individual or by family members;

PE.1.5.2 current emotional and behavioral functioning;

PE.1.5.3 maladaptive or problem behaviors;

PE.1.5.4 when indicated, a psychiatric evaluation;

PE.1.5.5 when indicated, a mental status examination appropriate to the individual's age;

PE.1.5.6 when indicated, a psychological assessment, including intellectual, projective, neuropsychological, and personality testing; and

PE.1.5.7 when indicated, other functional evaluations of language, self-care, visual-motor, and cognitive functioning.

PE.1.6 When indicated, assessments identify community resources used by the individual.

PE.1.7 A psychosocial assessment is completed and entered in the clinical record for each individual.

PE.1.7.1 As appropriate, the psychosocial assessment includes information about the individual's

PE.1.7.1.1 environment and home;

PE.1.7.1.2 leisure and recreation;

PE.1.7.1.3 religion and spiritual orientation;

PE.1.7.1.4 childhood history;

PE.1.7.1.5 military service history;

PE.1.7.1.6 financial status;

PE.1.7.1.7 usual social, peer-group, and environmental setting;

PE.1.7.1.8 sexual history and orientation; and

PE.1.7.1.9 family circumstances.

PE.1.7.2 The psychosocial assessment includes determining the need for the family's participation.

PE.1.7.3 In the care of a dying individual, the psychosocial assessment includes the social, spiritual, and cultural variables that influence the perceptions and expressions of grief by the individual or family.

PE.1.8 When appropriate, a vocational assessment is completed and entered in the clinical record.

PE.1.9 When appropriate, an educational assessment is completed and entered in the clinical record.

PE.1.10 When appropriate, a legal assessment is completed and entered in the clinical record.

PE.1.11 A physical health assessment, including a medical history and physical examination, is completed within 24 hours after admission to inpatient programs and within one week after admission to residential and therapeutic foster care programs.

PE.1.11.1 The physical health assessment consists of a medical history and, as indicated, a physical examination.

PE.1.11.2 In inpatient, residential, and therapeutic foster care programs serving children, adolescents, or developmentally disabled persons, the physical health assessment addresses

PE.1.11.2.1 motor development and functioning;

PE.1.11.2.2 sensorimotor functioning;

PE.1.11.2.3 speech, hearing, and language functioning;

PE.1.11.2.4 visual functioning;

PE.1.11.2.5 immunization status; and

PE.1.11.2.6 oral health and oral hygiene.

PE.1.12 All partial-hospitalization and outpatient programs comply with written procedures requiring a physical health screening to determine the need for a physical health assessment, including a medical history and physical examination.

PE.1.13 The organization has a written plan to ensure that medical histories, physical examinations, and laboratory tests not directly provided by the organization can be obtained when necessary.

PE.1.14 Diagnostic testing is performed to determine individuals' health care needs and as part of care.

PE.1.14.1 When the report of test results requires clinical interpretation, adequate clinical information is supplied with the request for the test.

PE.1.15 The scope and intensity of any further assessment are determined by the organization's mission and scope, the care setting, the individual's need and desire for care, and the individual's response to previous care.

PE.1.16 Pathology and clinical laboratory services and consultation are consistently and conveniently available to meet the needs of individuals served by the organization, as determined by the licensed independent practitioner(s) of the staff.

PE.1.16.1 Provision is made, either on the premises or through a reference or contract laboratory, for promptly performing adequate examinations in the fields of anatomic pathology, hematology, chemistry, microbiology, clinical microscopy, parasitology, immunohematology, serology, virology, and, as it relates to the pathology and clinical laboratory services, nuclear medicine.

PE.1.16.1.1 All laboratory testing performed while the individual is under the organization's care is done in the organization's laboratories (including the central laboratory and any ancillary, near-patient-testing, and point-of-care-testing laboratories) or in approved reference laboratories.

PE.1.16.1.2 The director(s) recommends reference laboratory services to the organization's leaders for acceptance through their designated mechanism.

PE.1.16.2 In the absence of organized central pathology and clinical laboratory services, the licensed independent practitioner(s) on staff establishes a mechanism for identifying acceptable reference and/or contract laboratory services.

PE.1.16.2.1 Reference and contract laboratory services meet applicable federal standards for clinical laboratories.

PE.1.16.3 The organization defines the extent to which waived test results are used in the provision of care to the individuals served (definitive or used only as a screen).

PE.1.16.3.1 The organization identifies the personnel responsible for performing and supervising waived testing.

PE.1.16.3.2 Personnel performing tests have adequate, specific training and orientation to perform the tests and demonstrate satisfactory levels of competence.

PE.1.16.3.3 Policies and procedures governing specific testing-related processes are current and readily available.

PE.1.16.3.4 Quality control checks, as defined by the organization, are conducted on each procedure.

PE.1.16.3.4.1 At a minimum, manufacturers' instructions are followed.

PE.1.16.3.5 Appropriate quality control and test records are maintained.

PE.1.17 A preanesthesia assessment is completed for each individual for whom anesthesia is contemplated.

PE.1.17.1 Each individual is reevaluated immediately before the induction of anesthesia.

PE.1.17.2 The individual's postprocedure status is assessed on admission to and discharge from the postanesthesia recovery area.

PE.1.18 Possible victims of abuse or neglect are identified using criteria developed by the organization.

PE.1.18.1 The organization's staff conducts the assessment of victims of alleged or suspected abuse or neglect or refers it to the appropriate setting.

PE.1.18.1.1 The assessment is conducted with the consent of the individual, parent, or legal guardian, or as otherwise provided by law.

PE.1.18.1.2 The assessment provides for collection, retention, and safeguarding of evidentiary material released by the individual.

PE.1.18.1.3 The assessment includes notification of the proper authorities and release of information, as required by law.

PE.1.19 Whenever services are provided to a child or an adolescent, family or guardian involvement is facilitated and coordinated throughout the assessment process.

PE.1.19.1 Services provided to a child or an adolescent include an assessment of the family's effect on the individual's condition and the effect of that condition on the family.

PE.1.19.2 Services provided to children and adolescents include assessing the individual's legal custody status, when applicable.

PE.1.19.3 Services provided to a child or an adolescent include assessing the individual's growth and development including physical, emotional, cognitive, educational, nutritional, and social development.

PE.1.19.4 Services provided to a child or an adolescent include assessing the individual's play and daily activities needs.

PE.1.19.5 Services provided to a child or an adolescent include assessing the family's or guardian's expectations for and involvement in the individual's assessment, initial treatment, and continuing care.

PE.1.20 Services provided to individuals with mental retardation or other developmental disabilities include a comprehensive assessment of the presenting problems, disabilities, needs, and, when possible, their causes.

PE.1.20.1 The comprehensive assessment of individuals with mental retardation and other developmental disabilities is conducted within 30 days of admission and at regular intervals thereafter.

PE.1.20.2 Services provided to individuals with mental retardation and other developmental disabilities include at least annual physical and dental examinations.

PE.1.20.3 Services provided to individuals with mental retardation and other developmental disabilities include at least annual assessments of physical development, developmental history, and health.

PE.1.20.4 A reassessment of social, emotional, behavioral, educational, vocational, and cognitive functioning, as well as recreational needs and, when appropriate, legal needs is conducted at regular intervals and at least annually for each individual.

PE.1.20.5 Admission to the program and provision of specific services are determined by the individual's needs and not solely by a court's determination of legal incompetence.

PE.1.20.6 The psychosocial assessment for individuals with mental retardation and other developmental disabilities addresses

PE.1.20.6.1 comprehensive social history;

PE.1.20.6.2 adaptive behavior, social functioning, and independent living skills; and

PE.1.20.6.3 skills, talents, aptitudes, interests, and leisure activities.

PE.1.20.7 The educational and vocational functioning assessment for individuals with mental retardation and other developmental disabilities addresses

PE.1.20.7.1 education and training history;

PE.1.20.7.2 work history; and

PE.1.20.7.3 work interests, skills, and work-related behavior.

PE.1.20.8 The cognitive functioning assessment for individuals with mental retardation and other developmental disabilities addresses

PE.1.20.8.1 intelligence testing;

PE.1.20.8.2 conceptual skills; and

PE.1.20.8.3 the current level of concrete and abstract reasoning.

PE.1.21 Assessment or reassessment of individuals receiving treatment for chemical dependency addresses

PE.1.21.1 history of alcohol, nicotine, and other drug use, including age of onset, duration, patterns of use, and consequences of use;

PE.1.21.2 history of physical problems associated with dependence;

PE.1.21.3 use of alcohol and other drugs by family members;

PE.1.21.4 religion and spiritual orientation;

PE.1.21.5 types of previous treatment and responses to that treatment; and

PE.1.21.6 any history of abuse.

PE.1.22 Discharge-planning needs are assessed.

PE.2 Assessment data are analyzed and integrated to identify and prioritize the individual's care needs.

PE.2.1 Care decisions are based on the individual's identified needs and care priorities.

PE.3 Each individual is reassessed at regularly specified times determined by the course of treatment.

PE.3.1 Each individual is reassessed to evaluate his or her response to treatment.

PE.3.2 Individuals are reassessed when significant changes occur in their condition.

PE.3.3 Individuals are reassessed when significant changes occur in their diagnosis.

PE.4 Activities required as part of assessment are defined in writing.

PE.4.1 Each discipline's scope of assessment is defined in writing.

PE.4.2 A qualified, clinically competent licensed independent practitioner is responsible for determining the degree of assessment and care for each individual treated in an emergency care area.

PE.4.3 A registered nurse assesses individuals' nursing care needs in all acute inpatient settings.

Standards and Intent Statements

Initial Screening and Clinical Assessments

Initial Screening

Standards

PE.1 *Each individual's physical and psychological status and social functioning are assessed.*

PE.1.1 An initial screening and/or assessment of each individual's physical, psychological, and social status is conducted to determine the need for care, the type of care to be provided, and the need for any further assessment.

Intent of PE.1 and PE.1.1

Information is gathered when individuals enter the setting or service to identify the reasons that bring them to the organization. The information to be collected is defined by the organization's policies and procedures and depends on the individual's emergent needs and the setting in which he or she seeks care. When appropriate, data from the individual's family are included.

Information gathered at the first contact can indicate the need for more data or a more intensive assessment of the individual's physical, psychological (including cognitive and communicative skills or development), or social functioning. The need for further assessment is determined, at least, by the treatment sought, the individual's presenting condition, and whether the individual agrees to treatment. The organization's policies and procedures address initial screening to determine the need for psychiatric evaluation and psychological testing. Policy also identifies what areas are included in reassessments.

Standard

PE.1.2 The organization has an assessment or screening procedure for the early detection of mental illness that is life threatening, indicates severe personality disorganization or deterioration, or may seriously affect the treatment or rehabilitation process.

Intent of PE.1.2

Early in the assessment or screening process following admission, each individual is evaluated for mental illness that indicates the need for additional assessments, referrals, exceptional supervision, or intervention. This evaluation also considers the ability of the treatment setting to provide appropriate care to meet the assessed needs.

Standards

PE.1.3 The need for assessing each individual's nutritional status is determined.

PE.1.4 The need for assessing the full range of each individual's functional status is determined.

PE.1.4.1 An assessment of physical functioning is performed for each individual referred for physical rehabilitation services.

Intent of PE.1.3 Through PE.1.4.1

The initial screening or assessment identifies individuals who are at moderate or high nutritional risk and need a nutritional assessment by a qualified dietitian or another qualified professional(s).

The initial screening or assessment may trigger referrals for functional assessments by qualified rehabilitation professionals.

Clinical Assessments

Standards

PE.1.5 *An emotional and behavioral assessment of each individual is completed and entered in the clinical record. The assessment includes at least a history of emotional, behavioral, and substance-abuse problems, their co-occurrence or treatment, including*

PE.1.5.1 use of alcohol and other drugs by the individual or by family members;

PE.1.5.2 current emotional and behavioral functioning;

PE.1.5.3 maladaptive or problem behaviors;

PE.1.5.4 when indicated, a psychiatric evaluation;

PE.1.5.5 when indicated, a mental status examination appropriate to the individual's age;

PE.1.5.6 when indicated, a psychological assessment, including intellectual, projective, neuropsychological, and personality testing; and

PE.1.5.7 when indicated, other functional evaluations of language, self-care, visual-motor, and cognitive functioning.

Intent of PE.1.5 Through PE.1.5.7

Assessment of each individual's emotional and behavioral functioning may be conducted by using a variety of assessment tools. It may include evaluations by multiple disciplines and vary according to individuals' ages and disabilities.

Regardless of the technique used, the emotional and behavioral assessment always addresses the individual's history of mental health or behavioral problems and the circumstances surrounding the current admission. Assessment documentation includes integrating the assessment findings by clinicians.

Standard

PE.1.6 When indicated, assessments identify community resources used by the individual.

Intent of PE.1.6

For certain populations, the assessment process includes early identification of community resources with which the individual is familiar and to whom the individual is known. Such populations include the severely and persistently mentally ill and severely and chronically disabled individuals. These community resources, such as community mental health centers, sheltered workshops, sheltered living, day treatment, or activity programs, may be used as informational, discharge-planning, and continuing-care resources.

Standard

PE.1.7 A psychosocial assessment is completed and entered in the clinical record for each individual.

Intent of PE.1.7

The scope of the psychosocial assessment is defined and reflects the population(s) served and types of services provided.

Standards

PE.1.7.1 *The psychosocial assessment includes information about the individual's*

PE.1.7.1.1 environment and home;

PE.1.7.1.2 leisure and recreation;

PE.1.7.1.3 religion and spiritual orientation;

PE.1.7.1.4 childhood history;

PE.1.7.1.5 military service history;

PE.1.7.1.6 financial status;

PE.1.7.1.7 usual social, peer-group, and environmental setting;

PE.1.7.1.8 sexual history and orientation; and

PE.1.7.1.9 family circumstances.

Intent of PE.1.7.1 Through PE.1.7.1.9

A thorough psychosocial assessment consists of several components, including the data specified above plus a clinical analysis of this data in relation to the current admission and need for treatment. Documentation by the individual or referral source may be used only when supplemented with the findings of a clinical interview. Age or clinical considerations may require an expanded psychosocial assessment. The individual's family circumstances include the constellation of the family group, the current living situation, and social, ethnic, cultural, emotional, and health factors.

Standard

PE.1.7.2 The psychosocial assessment includes determining the need for the family's* participation.

Intent of PE.1.7.2

Family members are considered at an early stage as potential sources of data about the individual. They are also considered resources in the treatment process, offering information about the individual and other support.

Standard

PE.1.7.3 In the care of a dying individual, the psychosocial assessment includes the social, spiritual, and cultural variables that influence the perceptions and expressions of grief by the individual or family.

Intent of PE.1.7.3

The special issues of impending death and the importance of the bereavement process for survivors call for specific and focused caring. When death and loss are approaching, special attention is given to those issues, cultural practices, beliefs, and variables that provide dignity, respect, support, and meaning to the individuals involved. Assessment of these issues, planning, and interventions are documented as part of the care provided.

Standards

PE.1.8 When appropriate, a vocational assessment is completed and entered in the clinical record.

PE.1.9 When appropriate, an educational assessment is completed and entered in the clinical record.

Intent of PE.1.8 and PE.1.9

When indicated by their condition at admission, individuals' vocational or educational needs are assessed. Such assessments are also conducted at any time during the course of treatment, particularly when changes in needs or condition occur.

Standard

PE.1.10 When appropriate, a legal assessment is completed and entered in the clinical record.

Intent of PE.1.10

Early in the assessment, screening regarding legal involvement is appropriate for all individuals, followed by a complete assessment as indicated. Determination of current legal involvement most frequently addresses divorce, child custody, and criminal charges including misdemeanors or bankruptcy.

---

* **family** The person(s) who plays a significant role in the member's life, which may include an individual(s) not legally related to the member. This person(s) is often referred to as a surrogate decision maker, if authorized to make care decisions for a member who loses decision-making capacity.

Standard

PE.1.11 A physical health assessment, including a medical history and physical examination, is completed within 24 hours after admission to inpatient programs and within one week after admission to residential and therapeutic foster care programs.

Note: *This standard applies to inpatient programs, residential programs, therapeutic foster care programs, and overnight crisis stabilization or other programs that house patients overnight.*

Intent of PE.1.11

This assessment is performed by a licensed independent practitioner, who is qualified and competent to do so, within 24 hours of admission to inpatient programs and within one week after admission to residential programs and therapeutic foster care settings. This time frame applies to weekend and holiday admissions as well as to weekdays. Some situations may occur in which medical needs require completion of a physical health assessment within a shorter time frame.

If a comprehensive medical history and physical examination have been completed within 30 days before admission to the organization, a durable, legible copy of this report may be used in the clinical record as the physical health assessment, but any subsequent changes must be recorded at the time of admission. A physical health assessment conducted before admission may be used as an assessment tool in care planning only when

- it includes a medical history and physical examination;
- it was conducted by a competent and qualified licensed independent practitioner within 30 days of the current course of treatment; and
- the individual's condition remains consistent with the results of that examination.

The organization has documentation showing that the information is current. In addition, by accepting such a health assessment, the organization attests to its accuracy, completeness, and relevancy to the current course of treatment. The organization may never abdicate this responsibility to referral sources or other mental health professionals.

Standard

PE.1.11.1 The physical health assessment consists of a medical history and, as indicated, a physical examination.

Intent of PE.1.11.1

When a physical health assessment is conducted, it includes a complete medical history. Information gathered includes known diseases and specific physical complaints; previous hospitalizations and operative procedures; medications being taken; family history of illness; physical abuse; infectious and communicable diseases; current and past history of substance abuse, including age of onset, duration, patterns, and consequences of use; and the types of and responses to previous treatment. Physical health questions raised by the medical history are addressed in the current physical examination.

Standards

PE.1.11.2 *In inpatient, residential, and therapeutic foster care programs serving children, adolescents, or developmentally disabled persons, the physical health assessment addresses*

PE.1.11.2.1 motor development and functioning;

PE.1.11.2.2 sensorimotor functioning;

PE.1.11.2.3 speech, hearing, and language functioning;

PE.1.11.2.4 visual functioning;

PE.1.11.2.5 immunization status; and

PE.1.11.2.6 oral health and oral hygiene.

Intent of PE.1.11.2 Through PE.1.11.2.6

For the settings and populations identified in PE.1.11.2, an expanded physical health assessment is conducted. At a minimum, the assessment screens for less-than-optimal functioning and facilitates timely, in-depth evaluation or immediate intervention when indicated.

Standard

PE.1.12 All partial-hospitalization and outpatient programs comply with written procedures requiring a physical health screening to determine the need for a physical health assessment, including a medical history and physical examination.

Intent of PE.1.12

Organizations providing non-24-hour care services, such as supportive living, case management, or assertive community treatment, have procedures governing physical health screening. The procedures specify the data to be collected, responsible staff, a time frame, and decision criteria for determining the need for a physical examination. A qualified and competent licensed independent practitioner participates in developing the physical health screening procedure.

Information to be addressed in the physical health screening of individuals receiving partial-hospitalization and outpatient care or services includes

- significant known diagnoses;
- significant known past treatment procedures;
- past and current diagnoses or problems;
- known adverse and allergic drug reactions; and
- currently and recently used medications.

(Also see the intent of IM.7 through IM.7.2.27.)

Standard

PE.1.13 The organization has a written plan to ensure that medical histories, physical examinations, and laboratory tests not directly provided by the organization can be obtained when necessary.

Intent of PE.1.13

Organizations that do not provide physical health assessments or laboratory tests arrange for such services to be provided by an outside source (that is, a recognized health care organization, laboratory, or qualified and competent licensed independent practitioner). A written plan describes how the organization gets medical histories, physical examinations, and laboratory services it doesn't provide directly. Agreements with outside sources address such issues as maximum time from request to service delivery, mechanisms for recording and reporting findings, quality of services, fees for services, and reimbursement agreements.

Standards

PE.1.14 Diagnostic testing is performed to determine individuals' health care needs and as part of care.

PE.1.14.1 When the report of test results requires clinical interpretation, adequate clinical information is supplied with the request for the test.

Intent of PE.1.14 and PE.1.14.1

Diagnostic testing includes laboratory and other invasive and noninvasive diagnostic and imaging procedures as well as psychological tests. It also includes appropriate use of laboratory, radiologic, electrodiagnostic, and other tests and imaging technologies integral to the physical, psychological, and social assessment of the individual. A qualified licensed independent practitioner determines which tests, if any, should be performed when the individual enters the program or service. Requests for diagnostic testing include enough information, in writing, to facilitate testing and interpreting results.

Standard

PE.1.15 The scope and intensity of any further assessment are determined by the organization's mission and scope, the care setting, the individual's need and desire for care, and the individual's response to previous care.

Intent of PE.1.15

When indicated by use of screening criteria or a change in condition, an individual's status is assessed or reassessed on a more detailed basis, as described in organization planning documents. The individual's response to any previous care should also be considered in the decision about initiating further reassessment of biopsychosocial needs. Finally, the individual's need and desire for continuing or terminating care or services is a factor in reassessment decisions.

Pathology and Clinical Laboratory Services—Waived Testing

For organizations that provide laboratory services of moderate or high complexity, the standards in the *Comprehensive Accreditation Manual for Pathology and Clinical Laboratory Services* (*CAMPCLS*) supersede all laboratory standards in this manual. However, if an organization provides only limited laboratory testing (waived testing or testing referred to other organizations), it should refer to the standards in this section for the necessary requirements.

If the organization is performing waived testing only, standards PE.1.16.3 through PE.1.16.3.5 will apply. If the organization performs moderate-complexity or high-complexity testing, it must meet applicable standards in the *CAMPCLS*.

Standards

PE.1.16 Pathology and clinical laboratory services and consultation are consistently and conveniently available to meet the needs of individuals served by the organization, as determined by the licensed independent practitioner(s)* of the staff.

PE.1.16.1 Provision is made, either on the premises or through a reference or contract laboratory, for promptly performing adequate examinations in the fields of anatomic pathology, hematology, chemistry, microbiology, clinical microscopy, parasitology, immunohematology, serology, virology, and, as it relates to the pathology and clinical laboratory services, nuclear medicine.

Intent of PE.1.16 and PE.1.16.1

The organization has a system for providing required laboratory services either on or off site. Laboratory services may be part of the organization's structure, provided by agreement with another organization, or both. The type of laboratory services provided is based on the population served, services offered, and the organization's staff needs. When laboratory results are required to diagnose or treat an individual with a critical health status, the service(s) provides timely results.

Standards

PE.1.16.1.1 All laboratory testing performed while the individual is under the organization's care is done in the organization's laboratories (including the central laboratory and any ancillary, near-patient-testing, and point-of-care-testing laboratories) or in approved reference laboratories.

PE.1.16.1.2 The director(s) recommends reference laboratory services to the organization's leaders for acceptance through their designated mechanism.

PE.1.16.2 In the absence of organized central pathology and clinical laboratory services, the licensed independent practitioner(s) on staff establishes a mechanism for identifying acceptable reference and/or contract laboratory services.

PE.1.16.2.1 Reference and contract laboratory services meet applicable federal standards for clinical laboratories.

Intent of PE.1.16.1.1 Through PE.1.16.2.1

The organization's laboratory or reference laboratory delivers the quality performance and accurate results necessary for clinical decision making. The mechanism for selecting reference or contract laboratories includes evaluating the laboratory's performance, acceptability, and compliance with federal standards.

---

* **licensed independent practitioner (LIP)** Any individual permitted by law and by the organization to provide care services without direction or supervision, within the scope of the individual's licensure or certification and in accordance with individually granted clinical privileges (these individuals may also be referred to by other terms such as "independent care provider"). In many behavioral health organizations, LIPs include physicians, psychologists, and social workers.

Waived Testing

Overview

Because tests classified as "waived" under federal law and regulation are used to diagnose, treat, or monitor individuals, the personnel performing them need to follow good laboratory practices. The goal of the waived testing function* is to provide a framework for establishing minimum requirements for quality control, responsibility for testing, personnel, and reporting results.

The following standards address the requirements that must be carried out when the organization performs waived testing procedures. Waived tests are those that

- meet the Clinical Laboratory Improvement Amendments of 1988 (CLIA '88) requirements to be classified as waived tests;
- are cleared by the Food and Drug Administration (FDA) for home use;
- use methodologies that are so simple and accurate as to make the likelihood of erroneous results negligible; or
- pose no risk of harm to the individual served if the test is performed incorrectly.

Tests are constantly being evaluated for inclusion with those defined as "waived."

Note: *Testing methods classified as waived testing are in compliance with PE.1.16. 3 through PE.1.16.3.5.*

Standard

PE.1.16.3 The organization defines the extent to which waived test results are used in the provision of care to the individuals served (definitive or used only as a screen).

Intent of PE.1.16.3

The organization defines whether the results of waived testing will be considered definitive for purposes of care and diagnosis or regarded as a screening tool, in which case they may be followed by confirmation testing. The organization assesses all waived testing it performs and specifies how each test will be used in diagnosis, care, and screening.

Standard

PE.1.16.3.1 The organization identifies the personnel responsible for performing and supervising waived testing.

Intent for PE.1.16.3.1

The organization identifies which staff members perform testing and which direct or supervise testing. These staff may be employees of the organization, contracted personnel, or employees of a contracted service.

Standard

PE.1.16.3.2 Personnel performing tests have adequate, specific training and orientation to perform the tests and demonstrate satisfactory levels of competence.

* **function** A goal-directed, interrelated series of processes, such as performance improvement or infection control.

Intent for PE.1.16.3.2

For waived tests to be done properly, the personnel performing them must be qualified to do so. Therefore, the organization sees that the following three elements are fulfilled:

- Personnel have had specific training in the tests, which may be acquired through the organization or other training programs, such as those provided by other health care organizations or by manufacturers;
- They have had orientation specific to the laboratory's needs; and
- They have shown current competence.

Skills are assessed at defined intervals, determined by the director or supervisor, based on the frequency that staff members perform tests and their technical backgrounds. The organization emphasizes skills testing for individuals who perform testing infrequently.

Organizations also consider the complexity of the test methodology and the consequences of an inaccurate result. Methods used to assess current skills can include

- performing a test on an unknown specimen;
- periodic observation of routine work by the supervisor or a delegate; and
- monitoring each user's quality control performance.

The organization evaluates and documents this information.

Standard

PE.1.16.3.3 Policies and procedures governing specific testing-related processes are current and readily available.

Intent of PE.1.16.3.3

Written policies and procedures address the following items:

a. Specimen collection;
b. Specimen preservation;
c. Instrument calibration;
d. Quality control and remedial action;
e. Equipment performance evaluation; and
f. Test performance.

The policies and procedures for each item apply to the specific organization. Referring to a manufacturer's manual is acceptable, if appropriate modifications have been made to tailor the manual's content to the organization. The policies and procedures are available to the person performing the test. If they are located in an office, the person performing the test has access to the office.

Standards

PE.1.16.3.4 Quality control checks, as defined by the organization, are conducted on each procedure.

PE.1.16.3.4.1 At a minimum, manufacturers' instructions are followed.

Intent of PE.1.16.3.4 and PE.1.16.3.4.1

The organization's quality control plan includes a quality control program for testing.

The plan specifies how procedures will be controlled for quality, establishes timetables, and explains the rationale for choice of procedures and timetables. The rationale is based on

- how the test is used;
- reagent stability;
- manufacturer's recommendations;
- the organization's experience with the test; and
- currently accepted guidelines.

Quality control requirements for glucose meter testing include two levels of control for each instrument on each day of testing.

Standard

PE.1.16.3.5 Appropriate quality control and test records are maintained.

Intent for PE.1.16.3.5

Quality control test results are documented and test results may be located in the clinical record. Quality control records, instrument problems, and individual results are correlated. A log or other record is maintained to determine annual volume, if required by other reporting agencies.

Assessment for Anesthesia

Standards

PE.1.17 A preanesthesia assessment is completed for each individual for whom anesthesia* is contemplated.

PE.1.17.1 Each individual is reevaluated immediately before the induction of anesthesia.

PE.1.17.2 The individual's postprocedure status is assessed on admission to and discharge from the postanesthesia recovery area.

Intent of PE.1.17 Through PE.1.17.2

The individual's status is assessed continuously throughout the procedure when anesthesia is used. Continuing individual assessment includes a preanesthesia assessment incorporating data collected during the assessment process(es). Before anesthesia is administered, the individual is determined to be an appropriate candidate for undergoing the planned anesthesia.

A licensed independent practitioner with appropriate clinical privileges determines whether the individual is an appropriate candidate for anesthesia based on the results of the preanesthesia assessment, which supplies information needed to

- plan the choice of anesthesia care;
- safely administer anesthesia; and
- interpret findings while monitoring the individual.

Anesthesia does not include local anesthetic agents.

---

* See the "Care" chapter of this manual for the scope of anesthesia to which these standards apply.

Assessment of Abuse and Neglect

Standard

PE.1.18 Possible victims of abuse or neglect are identified using criteria developed by the organization.

Intent of PE.1.18

Victims of alleged or suspected abuse or neglect may be admitted to the organization through various programs or services. Appropriate care cannot be provided unless suspected or alleged victims are identified and assessed. Established criteria are used throughout the organization to identify possible victims of abuse. These criteria address at least physical assault, rape or other sexual molestation, domestic abuse, abuse of elders and children, and neglect.

Staff are taught how to apply these criteria, and a list of private and public community agencies that provide or arrange for assessment and care of abuse victims is maintained to facilitate appropriate referrals.

Standards

PE.1.18.1 The organization's staff conducts the assessment of victims of alleged or suspected abuse or neglect or refers it to the appropriate setting.

Note: *PE.1.18.1.1 through PE.1.18.1.3 are scored only when the organization conducts the assessment.*

PE.1.18.1.1 The assessment is conducted with the consent of the individual, parent, or legal guardian, or as otherwise provided by law.

PE.1.18.1.2 The assessment provides for collection, retention, and safeguarding of evidentiary material released by the individual.

PE.1.18.1.3 The assessment includes notification of the proper authorities and release of information, as required by law.

Intent of PE.1.18.1 Through PE.1.18.1.3

Individuals who are possible victims of alleged or suspected abuse or neglect have special needs related to the assessment or referral process. Because information and evidentiary material(s) may be collected that could be used in future legal actions, the organization has specific and unique responsibilities for safeguarding such material(s).

Consistent with organization policy, documentation in the individual's clinical record addresses the items in the standards.

Special Assessment of Children and Adolescents

Standard

PE.1.19 Whenever services are provided to a child or an adolescent, family or guardian involvement is facilitated and coordinated throughout the assessment process.*

Intent of PE.1.19

Active participation by family members is essential throughout the treatment of children and adolescents. The organization establishes routine procedures that facilitate ongoing communication with family about their perceptions of the individual's needs and other issues. In conducting the assessment, the organization should distinguish between data provided by family or referral sources and data based on interaction with the individual.

Standard

PE.1.19.1 Services provided to a child or an adolescent include an assessment of the family's effect on the individual's condition and the effect of that condition on the family.

Intent of PE.1.19.1

The psychosocial assessment documented in each individual's record objectively

- reports the family history and current living situation;
- assesses the family dynamics and their impact on the individual's current needs;
- identifies areas that should be addressed in the care process; and
- evaluates family dynamics as a factor in discharge planning.

Standard

PE.1.19.2 Services provided to children and adolescents include assessing the individual's legal custody status, when applicable.

Intent of PE.1.19.2

Legal custody can be a critical element in planning and providing care and aftercare. Responsibility for legal custody must be established and documented in the clinical record for children and adolescents of divorced parents and in instances where legal restrictions affect parental decision-making responsibility. As part of the assessment process, the organization identifies the adult(s) who has legal custody. This may prevent conflicts during care or discharge planning that can be detrimental to the child or adolescent.

Standard

PE.1.19.3 Services provided to a child or an adolescent include assessing the individual's growth and development including physical, emotional, cognitive, educational, nutritional, and social development.

---

* When the term "individuals or their families" or a variation of it is used in this manual, it takes into consideration the rights of the individual served to exercise personal privacy by withholding consent for participation in care and service decisions of family members or significant others.

Intent of PE.1.19.3

The organization uses a developmental perspective in evaluating all aspects of the child's or adolescent's functioning. Evaluations include assessment of individuals in relation to normative development for their chronological age.

Standard

PE.1.19.4 Services provided to a child or an adolescent include assessing the individual's play and daily activities needs.

Intent of PE.1.19.4

Play and daily activities are essential to development. Assessment of the play and daily activities typically engaged in by a child or adolescent is a useful indication of their psychosocial development; therefore, it must be considered as an integral part of the assessment process. In addition, the planning of care and services must take into account the child's or adolescent's need to engage in play and other activities as a part of daily living and as a potential medium for therapeutic intervention.

Standard

PE.1.19.5 Services provided to a child or an adolescent include assessing the family's or guardian's expectations for and involvement in the individual's assessment, initial treatment, and continuing care.

Intent of PE.1.19.5

Families play a significant role in the treatment of children and adolescents. The family's expectations and the expectations of the organization regarding their roles must be clear so that treatment begins and proceeds with a common understanding of what role each will play in achieving treatment goals. Family contacts are documented and, whenever possible, are conducted in person and in the presence of the child or adolescent.

Special Assessment of Individuals with Mental Retardation or Other Developmental Disabilities (MR/DD)

Standard

PE.1.20 Services provided to individuals with mental retardation or other developmental disabilities include a comprehensive assessment of the presenting problems, disabilities, needs, and, when possible, their causes.

Intent of PE.1.20

The organization establishes a comprehensive assessment to identify the needs of all individuals with mental retardation or other developmental disabilities. The assessment, shaped by the principle of normalization, reflects a historical perspective that takes into account both previous and current functioning.

Standards

PE.1.20.1 The comprehensive assessment of individuals with mental retardation and other developmental disabilities is conducted within 30 days of admission and at regular intervals thereafter.

PE.1.20.2 Services provided to individuals with mental retardation and other developmental disabilities include at least annual physical and dental examinations.

PE.1.20.3 Services provided to individuals with mental retardation and other developmental disabilities include at least annual assessments of physical development, developmental history, and health.

PE.1.20.4 A reassessment of social, emotional, behavioral, educational, vocational, and cognitive functioning, as well as recreational needs and, when appropriate, legal needs is conducted at regular intervals and at least annually for each individual.

Intent of PE.1.20.1 Through PE.1.20.4

Persons with mental retardation and other developmental disabilities are at risk for complex health, sensory, motor, and developmental problems. Minimal parameters for the timeliness of assessments are identified. Such assessments should facilitate timely intervention, when indicated. Reassessments are conducted whenever more current information is needed. The organization identifies the most common instances in which a reassessment should be done more often than once a year.

Standard

PE.1.20.5 Admission to the program and provision of specific services are determined by the individual's needs and not solely by a court's determination of legal incompetence.

Intent of PE.1.20.5

Admission policies are based on a match between the individual's identified needs and the organization's capability to provide needed services.

Standards

PE.1.20.6 *The psychosocial assessment for individuals with mental retardation and other developmental disabilities addresses*

PE.1.20.6.1 comprehensive social history;

PE.1.20.6.2 adaptive behavior, social functioning, and independent living skills; and

PE.1.20.6.3 skills, talents, aptitudes, interests, and leisure activities.

Intent of PE.1.20.6 Through PE.1.20.6.3

The preceding standards outline essential components of any thorough assessment of psychosocial functioning. In addition, the assessment of social functioning includes a clinical evaluation of the implications of assessment findings for developing an individual program plan. The assessment should distinguish between data provided by family or referral sources and data based on interaction with the individual.

Standards

PE.1.20.7 *The educational and vocational functioning assessment for individuals with mental retardation and other developmental disabilities addresses*

PE.1.20.7.1 education and training history;

PE.1.20.7.2 work history; and

PE.1.20.7.3 work interests, skills, and work-related behavior.

Intent of PE.1.20.7 Through PE.1.20.7.3

The organization defines the scope of the assessment of educational and vocational functioning to be completed for each individual served. The assessment involves collecting information about all three areas in the preceding standards. The depth of each individual assessment is appropriate to the individual's level of cognitive functioning.

Standards

PE.1.20.8 *The cognitive functioning assessment for individuals with mental retardation and other developmental disabilities addresses*

PE.1.20.8.1 intelligence testing;

PE.1.20.8.2 conceptual skills; and

PE.1.20.8.3 the current level of concrete and abstract reasoning.

Intent of PE.1.20.8 Through PE.1.20.8.3

A thorough assessment of cognitive functioning includes a quantitative evaluation of intellectual functioning as well as a qualitative assessment of the individual's concrete and abstract reasoning skills. The results of the assessment should be taken into consideration when selecting individual program plan interventions and objectives.

Special Assessment of Individuals in Chemical Dependency Programs and Services

Standards

PE.1.21 *Assessment or reassessment of individuals receiving treatment for chemical dependency addresses*

PE.1.21.1 history of alcohol, nicotine, and other drug use, including age of onset, duration, patterns of use, and consequences of use;

PE.1.21.2 history of physical problems associated with dependence;

PE.1.21.3 use of alcohol and other drugs by family members;

PE.1.21.4 religion and spiritual orientation;

PE.1.21.5 types of previous treatment and responses to that treatment; and

PE.1.21.6 any history of abuse.

Intent of PE.1.21 Through PE.1.21.6

Obtaining and interpreting information about substance abuse is necessary to develop treatment plans. By getting the data/information on the items listed in the standards, the clinician can

- assess the relationship of the physical state of each individual to the dependence;
- assess the nature of the individual's compulsion to use alcohol or other drugs;
- assess the intensity of the individual's mental preoccupation with using alcohol or drugs;
- distinguish between alcohol-related and other drug-related symptoms and other preexisting physical problems or pathologic behaviors; and
- establish a predictive value for success of treatment.

Factors assessed and considered in providing services to the individual served include

- obtaining a history of mental, emotional, and behavioral problems; their co-occurrences with substance use problems; and their treatment.
- identifying the physical, emotional, behavioral, and social functioning of the individual before the onset of chemical dependency.
- evaluating the effects that chemical dependency has had on each individual's physical, emotional, and social well-being.
- evaluating patterns of use, for example, continuous, episodic, or binge use.
- identifying consequences of use, for example, legal problems, divorce, loss of friends, job-related incidents, financial difficulties, blackouts, memory impairment.
- assessing the history of physical problems associated with chemical dependency to help substantiate the diagnosis, to anticipate potential medical problems related to chemical withdrawal management, to identify the individual's level of function, and to help the individual who is minimizing the physical consequences of dependence.
- assessing information about the use of alcohol or other drugs by the family to enhance understanding of the individual's behavioral dynamics and help determine the potential for extended family support, as well as the impact of family circumstances on treatment.
- assessing each individual's spiritual orientation, which may relate to the dependency in terms of how the individual views himself/herself as an individual of value and worth. Spiritual orientation is not considered synonymous with an individual's relationship with an organized religion.
- assessing any previous treatment and response to the treatment to see whether the individual responded appropriately to the treatment and if expected outcomes were achieved. If not, what revisions were made, if any?
- assessing whether the individual has experienced a history of abuse (including physical or sexual abuse either as the abuser or the abused) that may affect the individual's ability to address his or her dependence.

Assessment for Discharge-Planning Care Decisions and Reassessment

Standard

PE.1.22 Discharge-planning needs are assessed.

Intent of PE.1.22

To facilitate timely, appropriate, and continuous post-discharge care, assessments are conducted to support discharge planning. When indicated, this planning begins when the individual enters the setting. Discharge planning is most effective when related assessment processes are established and consistently used.

Standards

PE.2 Assessment data are analyzed and integrated to identify and prioritize the individual's care needs.

PE.2.1 Care decisions are based on the individual's identified needs and care priorities.

Intent of PE.2 and PE.2.1

An individual's primary health care professional and various other care providers may perform assessments of the individual. The data gathered in performing these assessments, the analysis of these data, and the subsequent integration of information about the individual facilitate identifying and prioritizing the individual's needs and help to determine the care and services to be provided.

Care decisions are based on individual needs identified through analyzing assessment data. For example, appropriate professional interventions are performed when variations in the individual's status are identified.

Reassessment

Standards

PE.3 Each individual is reassessed at regularly specified times determined by the course of treatment.

PE.3.1 Each individual is reassessed to evaluate his or her response to treatment.

PE.3.2 Individuals are reassessed when significant changes occur in their condition.

PE.3.3 Individuals are reassessed when significant changes occur in their diagnosis.

Intent of PE.3 Through PE.3.3

To ensure that care decisions continue to be appropriate, each individual's status is periodically reviewed. This review process is ongoing throughout the individual's contact with the organization and is triggered at key decision points as well as at intervals specified by the organization. The content of the review process and the interval between assessments is defined in organization planning documents.

Reassessment of individuals receiving treatment for alcoholism or other drug dependence considers the impact of major life changes on their treatment. The reassessment addresses the long-term and short-term effectiveness of specific services provided to meet the individual's needs.

Informed decision making is based on regular reassessment using mutually agreeable and reliable measures of the individual's choices, goals, strengths, symptoms, and behavioral patterns.

Structures Supporting the Assessment Process

Standards

PE.4 Activities required as part of assessment are defined in writing.

PE.4.1 Each discipline's scope of assessment is defined in writing.

Intent of PE.4 and PE.4.1

To provide consistent assessment of individual needs, the organization defines in writing the scope of assessments to be performed by each clinical discipline consistent with its scope of practice, state licensure laws, applicable regulations, certification, or registration. For example, the organization determines the applicable law or regulation governing who may perform nutritional assessments.

Assessment activities are defined in planning documents (that is, policies and procedures, protocols, or other such documented guidelines) that specify

- the data gathered to assess individual needs;
- the scope of assessment by each discipline;
- how data are analyzed to select an approach to meeting individual care needs; and
- the framework for decision making based on the analysis of assessment information.

Standard

PE.4.2 A qualified, clinically competent licensed independent practitioner is responsible for determining the degree of assessment and care for each individual treated in an emergency care area.

Intent of PE.4.2

Because the need for immediate care is usually greatest for individuals in the emergency care area, the intensity and scope of medical and psychological assessments done in the emergency care area are determined by a clinically competent professional who is qualified under applicable licensure, laws, regulations, registration, or certification.

Standard

PE.4.3 A registered nurse assesses individuals' nursing care needs in all acute* inpatient settings.

* Acute may also include crisis stabilization, medical detoxification, etc.

Intent of PE.4.3

In accordance with organization policy, a registered nurse determines and prioritizes the individual's nursing care needs at the time of initial assessment in inpatient settings. These activities require the judgment and skill of a registered nurse. Acute inpatient programs have a registered nurse on duty at all times to plan, assign, supervise, and evaluate nursing care and to provide delivery of nursing care to individuals served. Other qualified nursing staff members, such as licensed practical/vocational nurses, mental health technicians, or nursing assistants can assist the registered nurse during any aspect of the assessment process. Delegated assessment activities are performed in accordance with applicable law and regulation, and organization policies and procedures.

Care

Overview

The **goal** of the care function* is to provide individualized, planned, and appropriate interventions. "Care" includes care, treatment, services, rehabilitation, habilitation, or another intervention for the individual served by the organization. Care is given in settings that meet individuals' needs and enable them to reach care, treatment, rehabilitation, or habilitation goals.

Rehabilitation and habilitation refer to care and services designed to help individuals regain or achieve their optimal level of functioning, self-care, self-responsibility, independence, and quality of life. Their purpose is to minimize symptoms, exacerbation of chronic illness, impairments, and disabilities.

All interventions encourage individuals to make choices, maintain a sense of achievement about treatment progress, and continue or modify participation in care, treatment, and rehabilitation.

The assessment process, as described in the "Assessment" chapter of this manual (page 61), identifies the individual's physical, cognitive, behavioral, emotional, and social status. This assessment identifies facilitating factors and possible barriers to the individual reaching his or her goals beyond the presenting problems, for example,

- substance-use disorders;
- emotional, behavioral, and mental disorders;
- cognitive disorders;
- communicative disorders;
- developmental disabilities;
- vision and hearing impairments and disabilities;
- physical disabilities; and
- social and environmental factors.

The assessment process also helps determine the type of program or care or service activities and accommodations that will increase the individual's readiness to use the rehabilitation care and services.

To deliver effective care and services, the following key processes must be performed well:

- **Formulating, maintaining, and supporting an individual-specific treatment plan.**† The plan is developed based on individual needs identified through assessment.‡ The plan specifies individual goals and objectives, as well as the actions or interventions needed to meet them. Individuals agree to the planned course of treatment.§ A rehabilitation or habilitation plan describes a strategy for providing the specific skills and supports that will enable the individual to function in an environment that optimizes independence and choice while minimizing supervision and restrictiveness. Specific criteria are defined for the transition to more independent and less restrictive environments and integration into natural community settings. Rehabilitation offers

* **function** A goal-directed, interrelated series of processes, such as assessment or care of the individual.

† **treatment plan** A plan, based on data gathered during the assessment, that identifies the individual's care needs, lists the strategy for providing services to meet those needs, documents treatment goals and objectives, and outlines the criteria for terminating specified interventions. The format of the "plan" in some organizations may be guided by individual-specific policies and procedures, protocols, practice guidelines, clinical paths, or a combination of several methods.

‡ As described in the "Assessment" chapter of this manual.

§ See the "Rights, Responsibilities, and Ethics" chapter of this manual.

access to community resources and services that promote continued goal achievement and independence after the rehabilitation program concludes.

- **Implementation of the treatment plan.** Planned actions or interventions are carried out by staff in accordance with organization policy and procedure, standards of practice, and authorized scope of practice. Some interventions may also be performed by the individual, family,* or other caregiver following appropriate education.
- **Monitoring response to care and services.** Individuals are monitored and reassessed to determine the effectiveness of actions or interventions in meeting goals.
- **Modification of the treatment plan.** Care may be modified or terminated based on reassessment, the individual's need for further care, and achievement of treatment plan goals. Reassessment may result in the individual's transfer to another setting or service or discharge from the organization. Rehabilitation decision making is based on regular reassessment and reliable measures of the individual's needs, strengths, symptoms, behavioral patterns, and goal achievement. Care choices should be mutually agreeable to the individual and clinician.
- **Coordination of continuing care and services.** Continuing care, treatment, services, rehabilitation, habilitation, or other programs are planned and coordinated to meet the individual's needs after discharge.†

The activities described above will be performed by a variety of clinicians whose roles and responsibilities are determined by the component of care or service being provided, relevant licensure, law and regulation, registration, certification, privileges, scope of practice, or job description.

All interventions respect and encourage the individual to develop and maintain a sense of achievement and make choices about participation in care and services.

These standards do not prescribe a particular structure or method for performing these processes.

Note: *The first set of standards in this chapter, under treatment planning, outlines a process common to all individuals served receiving care and services and addresses the core processes (that is, planning, providing, monitoring); thus, it applies to every organization. Succeeding standards (Program Plans for Individuals with Mental Retardation and Other Developmental Disabilities through Anesthesia Care) address issues specific to certain types of care and service. Each standard or group of standards in these sections apply only when an organization provides the type of care or service addressed by the standard(s).*

---

* **family** The person(s) who plays a significant role in the member's life, which may include an individual(s) not legally related to the member. This person(s) is often referred to as a surrogate decision maker, if authorized to make care decisions for a member who loses decision-making capacity.

† See the "Continuum" chapter of this manual.

Standards

A list of all standards for this function appears below, presented without footnotes or other explanatory text. If you have any questions about a term used here, please refer to the standard as it appears in the next section of this chapter—Standards and Intent Statements.

TX.1 Treatment planning identifies care and services appropriate to the individual's specific needs and the severity of condition, impairment, or disability.

TX.1.1 Appropriate therapeutic efforts may begin before a full treatment plan is formulated.

TX.1.2 A preliminary treatment plan is developed based on an initial screening and is refined in response to additional clinical information.

TX.1.3 Qualified and competent individuals plan and provide care and services specific to the individual's needs and, as appropriate to the care and services given, in a collaborative and interdisciplinary manner.

TX.1.4 The treatment plan reflects the organization's treatment philosophy.

TX.1.5 The treatment plan reflects the individual's clinical needs, condition, functional strengths, and limitations.

TX.1.5.1 Rehabilitation services address assessed needs, in accordance with an individualized written plan of care developed by qualified and competent individuals.

TX.1.5.2 Justification is documented when identified needs are not addressed.

TX.1.5.3 Individuals' perceptions of their needs are documented, as are the families' perceptions when appropriate and available.

TX.1.5.4 Individuals are encouraged to participate in developing their treatment plans, and their involvement is documented.

TX.1.5.5 The treatment plan addresses the involvement of family when indicated.

TX.1.5.6 The treatment plan includes advocacy services when indicated to enhance the natural support system, facilitate environmental modifications, or create new supports.

TX.1.6 The treatment plan contains specific goals for achieving emotional and/or physical health as well as maximum growth and adaptive capabilities.

TX.1.6.1 Treatment-plan goals are based on assessments of the individual and, as appropriate, the family.

TX.1.6.2 Treatment-plan goals are linked to living, learning, and work activities.

TX.1.7 The treatment plan includes specific objectives for the goals identified in the plan.

TX.1.7.1 Rehabilitation plans include a description of facilitating factors and possible barriers to using rehabilitation services or reaching rehabilitation goals.

TX.1.8 The treatment plan specifies the interventions and approaches necessary to meet the individual's needs and goals.

TX.1.8.1 When the individual's identified needs include developing skills for activities of daily living, a training program is developed.

TX.1.8.2 Activity services, when provided, are incorporated into the treatment plan to provide a consistent and well-structured framework.

TX.1.8.3 The treatment plan includes specialized rehabilitation services to restore or maintain the functional abilities of individuals with physical, cognitive, social, leisure, or sensoriperceptual impairments, or whose primary problem is mental illness.

TX.1.8.4 When individuals need services not offered by the organization, appropriate referrals are made and documented in the clinical record.

TX.1.9 The treatment plan specifies the frequency of treatment procedures.

TX.1.10 Goals are periodically evaluated and, when necessary, revised, based on reassessment of the individual's current clinical problems, needs, and responses to treatment.

TX.1.11 The treatment plan stipulates specific criteria for discharge or terminating treatment.

TX.1.12 In inpatient and residential programs, the organization's oral health program has mechanisms designed to meet individuals' oral health care needs. The objectives and scope of the oral health program include at least

TX.1.12.1 in keeping with length of stay, the method(s) of providing, or referring individuals for, regular dental care;

TX.1.12.2 the method(s) of providing emergency dental care;

TX.1.12.3 daily oral hygiene procedures, including cleaning individuals' prostheses; and

TX.1.12.4 the proper labeling and storage of individuals' oral hygiene supplies and prostheses.

TX.1.13 Organization policy promotes access to appropriate educational services for each child or adolescent whose treatment causes a significant absence from school.

TX.1.13.1 Educational services are designed to meet the child's or adolescent's treatment needs and provide educational continuity.

TX.1.14 Programs offering services to individuals with mental retardation and other developmental disabilities accept and implement the principle of normalization.

TX.1.15 A behavior management team develops an individualized program within 30 days of admission which it reviews and revises at key decision points, or at least annually.

TX.1.15.1 The plan is reviewed upon admission, transfer, and discharge and is revised as necessary.

TX.1.15.2 The plan is reviewed when major changes occur in presenting problems or disabilities and is revised as necessary.

TX.1.15.3 The plan is reviewed when introducing protective devices or aversive consequences to address maladaptive behavior and is revised as necessary.

TX.1.15.4 The plan is reviewed when the individual reaches majority or emancipation and is revised as necessary.

TX.1.15.4.1 When individuals reach majority or emancipation, their civil and legal rights and, when appropriate, need for continued care or services are re-evaluated.

TX.1.16 Individuals or family members or advocates participate in individualized program planning, and their opinions and preferences about services, activities, and objectives are considered.

TX.1.16.1 Inability or unwillingness to participate in program planning is documented in the clinical record.

TX.1.17 When indicated to meet specified objectives, the clinical record addresses the use of corrective, adaptive, and prosthetic supports or devices and describes

TX.1.17.1 the reason for their use; and

TX.1.17.2 how often and under what circumstances they will be used.

TX.1.18 When indicated to meet a specified objective, the clinical record addresses using training programs for activities of daily living (ADLs) and describes

TX.1.18.1 the reason for such a program;

TX.1.18.2 how often and under what circumstances program activities will be conducted; and

TX.1.18.3 the methods to be used.

TX.1.19 When indicated to meet a specified objective, the individual program plan addresses the use of behavior-management procedures and describes

TX.1.19.1 the reason for such procedures;

TX.1.19.2 the methods to be used;

TX.1.19.3 how often or under what circumstances they will be used; and

TX.1.19.4 any restriction of the individual's rights.

TX.1.20 The organization provides for the health maintenance of all individuals served, including early detection and remediation of health needs.

TX.1.20.1 Each individual's height is recorded in the clinical record.

TX.1.20.2 When appropriate, an individual's weight is recorded in the clinical record at least quarterly.

TX.1.20.3 The organization provides for corrective, adaptive, and prosthetic devices in accordance with assessment findings.

TX.1.20.4 The organization implements written policies and procedures concerning detection of injury, disease, neglect, and abuse.

TX.1.20.5 Seizure activity and periodic determination of anticonvulsant drug levels are accurately recorded in the individual's clinical record when indicated.

TX.1.20.6 When physical therapy services are provided, they are supervised and coordinated by a qualified physical therapist.

TX.2 Systems and processes are implemented for the safe and effective use of medication.

TX.2.1 The organization identifies an appropriate selection of medications available for prescription or ordering.

TX.2.1.1 The organization establishes procedures for prescribing or ordering and procuring medications not available in the organization.

TX.2.1.2 Policies and procedures support safe prescription or ordering practices.

TX.2.2 The preparation, dispensing, and storage of medications adhere to law, regulation, licensure, and professional standards of practice.

TX.2.2.1 Medications are appropriately controlled during preparation and dispensing.

TX.2.2.2 If the organization prepares, dispenses, or stores medications, a medication-dose system is followed.

TX.2.2.3 A pharmacist reviews all prescriptions or orders.

TX.2.2.4 Important individual medication information is captured, communicated, and considered when preparing and dispensing medications.

TX.2.2.5 Pharmacy services are available when the organization's pharmacy service is closed or not available or when access to medications is limited.

TX.2.2.6 Emergency medication systems are available, when appropriate.

TX.2.2.7 A medication-recall system provides for retrieval and safe disposition of discontinued, expired, and recalled medications.

TX.2.3 Prescriptions or orders are verified and individuals are identified before medications are administered.

TX.2.3.1 Qualified individuals administer medications.

TX.2.3.2 Systems are implemented to support self-administration or alternative medication administration systems.

TX.2.3.3 Investigational medications are safely controlled and administered.

TX.2.4 Medication's effect on the individual is monitored continuously.

TX.2.4.1 Effects of medication are assessed based on information maintained in the individual's clinical record and medication profile and observations by staff and the individual.

TX.3 Designated special treatment procedures require clinical justification.

TX.3.1 Restraint or seclusion use within the organization is limited to those situations with adequate, appropriate clinical justification.

TX.3.1.1 Organization leaders support limited, justified use of restraint or seclusion through the following:

TX.3.1.1.1 Plans, policies, and priorities;

TX.3.1.1.2 Human resource planning;

TX.3.1.1.3 Staff orientation and education that creates a culture emphasizing prevention and appropriate use and encouraging alternatives;

TX.3.1.1.4 Education of the individual and, when appropriate, his or her family;

TX.3.1.1.5 Assessment processes that identify and, when appropriate, prevent potential behavioral risk factors;

TX.3.1.1.6 Design and delivery of care; and

TX.3.1.1.7 The development and promotion of preventive strategies and use of safe and effective alternatives.

TX.3.1.2 Performance-improvement processes identify opportunities, when appropriate, to reduce restraint or seclusion use.

TX.3.1.3 When restraint or seclusion is used, organization policy and procedures guide appropriate and safe use.

TX.3.1.3.1 Protocols that guide using restraint as an integral component of medical, dental, diagnostic, or surgical procedures or devices are consistent with organization policy.

TX.3.1.3.1.1 The appropriate clinical staff approve the protocols.

TX.3.1.3.1.2 Criteria are used to select individuals for care under the protocol.

TX.3.1.3.1.3 Qualified staff are identified and permitted to apply the criteria.

TX.3.1.3.2 Individual orders for restraint or seclusion are consistent with organization policy.

TX.3.1.3.2.1 Individuals' rights, dignity, and well-being are protected during restraint or seclusion use.

TX.3.1.3.2.2 Restraint or seclusion use is based on the assessed needs of the individual.

TX.3.1.3.2.3 The least restrictive, safe, and effective restraint or seclusion method is used.

TX.3.1.3.2.4 Restraint or seclusion is used correctly by competent, trained staff.

TX.3.1.3.2.5 Individuals in restraint or seclusion are monitored and reassessed appropriately.

TX.3.1.3.2.6 The needs of the individual are met during restraint or seclusion use.

TX.3.1.3.2.7 Restraint or seclusion use is ordered by a licensed independent practitioner.

TX.3.1.3.2.8 Orders for restraint or seclusion define specific time limits.

TX.3.1.3.3 Documentation in clinical records reflects organization policy.

TX.3.2 Policies and procedures govern the use of electroconvulsive therapy and other forms of convulsive therapy.

TX.3.2.1 Written consent for any use of electroconvulsive therapy or other forms of convulsive therapy is obtained from the individual and documented in the clinical record.

TX.3.3 Policies and procedures govern the use of unusual medications and investigational and experimental drugs.

TX.3.3.1 Investigational drugs are used only under the principal investigator's supervision and with the approval of the physician members of the clinical staff or an appropriate clinical staff committee, the research review committee, and appropriate federal, state, and local agencies.

TX.3.4 Policies and procedures govern maintenance use of drugs that have abuse potential (usually considered to be controlled substances and drugs which can be used as chemical restraints), are known to involve substantial risk, or are associated with significant, undesirable side effects.

TX.3.4.1 The organization's list of selected medications includes prescribed and administered maintenance drugs that have abuse potential.

TX.3.5 Policies and procedures govern the use of behavior management procedures for controlling maladaptive or problem behavior.

TX.3.5.1 The organization requires a positive approach to behavior management and the progressive use of the least restrictive alternatives.

TX.3.5.2 The clinical leaders specify and approve the behavior management procedures that can be used in the organization.

TX.3.5.3 Behavior management programs identify and teach the individual appropriate expression of the target behavior or alternative adaptive behaviors.

TX.3.5.4 Procedures that may result in denying a nutritionally adequate diet are prohibited.

TX.3.5.5 Seclusion other than in accordance with standards in this chapter is prohibited.

TX.3.5.6 Corporal punishment is prohibited.

TX.3.5.7 Fear-eliciting procedures are prohibited.

TX.3.5.8 Other individuals served by the organization's services are prohibited from carrying out an individual's behavior management program.

TX.3.5.9 A behavior management committee established by the clinical staff reviews, evaluates, and approves all behavior management programs.

TX.3.5.10 Time-out is used in accordance with the individual's program plan and the organization's policies and procedures.

TX.3.5.11 Aversive behavioral consequences are used only when withholding this intervention would be contrary to the individual's best interests and less restrictive alternatives have failed.

TX.3.5.12 Aversive behavioral consequences for maladaptive behavior are used in accordance with the individual's behavior management plan and organization policies and procedures.

TX.3.6 Legal, correctional, and/or administrative decisions affecting an individual's treatment are coordinated with clinical decisions, including those related to

TX.3.6.1 use of seclusion and restraint for nonclinical purposes;

TX.3.6.2 imposition of disciplinary restrictions;

TX.3.6.3 length of stay;

TX.3.6.4 restriction of rights; and

TX.3.6.5 plan for discharge and continuing care.

TX.4 The plan for nutrition care is developed and, when necessary, revised through a process whenever appropriate to the individual served.

TX.4.1 Authorized individuals prescribe or order nutrition care in a timely manner.

TX.4.2 The organization defines and assigns responsibility for preparing, storing, distributing, and administering food and nutrition therapy products.

TX.4.3 Food and nutrition therapy products are distributed and administered in a safe, accurate, and timely manner to the individual for whom they were prescribed or ordered.

TX.4.4 The organization has a process for providing food or nutrition therapy when diets or diet schedules are altered.

TX.4.5 Each individual is monitored for the nutrition's effectiveness and appropriateness.

TX.4.6 Nutrition care approaches and processes are standardized and communicated throughout the organization.

TX.5 An initial physical therapy evaluation and assessment are conducted before physical therapy services are provided.

TX.5.1 Whenever physical therapy is provided, treatment goals and plans are developed that are consistent with the diagnosis, the prognosis, and the aim of preventing or reducing disability or pain and restoring lost function.

TX.5.2 Whenever physical therapy is provided, planned services include therapeutic interventions that enhance daily living.

TX.5.3 Physical therapy staff monitor the extent to which services have met the therapeutic goals established through assessments, caused improvement of the identified physical dysfunction, or reduced pain associated with movement.

TX.6 A preanesthesia assessment is completed before anesthesia is administered.

TX.6.1 A plan for anesthesia care is developed.

TX.6.2 Anesthesia options and risks are addressed with the individual and family, if appropriate.

TX.6.3 The individual's physiological and neurological status is measured and assessed during the administration of anesthesia.

TX.6.4 The individual's postprocedure status is assessed on admission to and before discharge from the postanesthesia recovery area or the setting.

TX.6.4.1 Individuals are discharged from the recovery area by a qualified licensed independent practitioner or according to approved criteria.

TX.6.4.1.1 When discharge criteria are used, compliance with the criteria is fully documented in the individual's clinical record.

Standards and Intent Statements

Treatment Planning

Standard

TX.1 Treatment planning* identifies care and services appropriate to the individual's specific needs and the severity of condition, impairment, or disability.

Intent of TX.1

Delivering care and services effectively and efficiently requires planning. The treatment-planning process is designed to identify and incorporate each individual's unique needs, expectations, and characteristics into an individualized and appropriate plan. The nature of the individual's needs and condition, as determined through assessment, is a primary consideration during the planning process.

Standard

TX.1.1 Appropriate therapeutic efforts may begin before a full treatment plan is formulated.

Intent of TX.1.1

Care is provided in response to identified individual needs on a timely basis. For needs that are emergent or immediately apparent (such as clinical, psychiatric, or behavioral instability), a preliminary treatment plan is formulated and interventions carried out while full detailed assessments are underway. Assessment, reassessment, and care are dynamic, ongoing processes often performed concurrently.

Standard

TX.1.2 A preliminary treatment plan is developed based on an initial screening and is refined in response to additional clinical information.

Intent of TX.1.2

The treatment-planning process proceeds with the assessment process. A preliminary plan is developed as soon as possible, based on clinical information gathered during admission and initial assessment. Early initial planning is particularly important in identifying interventions to respond to emergency needs, such as a suicidal crisis, other dangers to self or others, or severe personality disorganization.

Standard

TX.1.3 Qualified and competent individuals† plan and provide care and services specific to the individual's needs and, as appropriate to the care and services given, in a collaborative and interdisciplinary manner.

---

* The term "treatment planning" includes care planning, individual program planning, habilitation planning, and rehabilitation planning.

† **qualified and competent individual or staff** An individual or staff member who is qualified to participate in one or all of the mechanisms outlined in the standards by virtue of the following: education, training, experience, competence, applicable licensure, law and regulation, registration, and/or certification.

Intent of TX.1.3

When appropriate to the services provided, collaborative and interdisciplinary care planning and delivery facilitate responsiveness to individual needs, achievement of care goals, and optimal outcomes. Care and services provided are always appropriate to individuals' identified needs. The mix of disciplines involved in care depends on the services provided, and the intensity of collaboration varies according to each individual's needs. Services are provided by qualified rehabilitation professionals whom the organization has determined to be competent by education, licensure, registration, certification, training, or experience.

Standard

TX.1.4 The treatment plan reflects the organization's treatment philosophy.

Intent of TX.1.4

Developing, adapting, or adopting a treatment philosophy is the basis for an organizational approach to providing care and services. Treatment planning and service delivery are consistent with the organization's defined treatment philosophy.

Standard

TX.1.5 The treatment plan reflects the individual's clinical needs, condition, functional strengths, and limitations.

Intent of TX.1.5

Treatment planning is a dynamic and flexible process that responds to continuing assessment of individual needs and status. It identifies the individual's functional* strengths and limitations and, as appropriate, relates them to the individual's needs. The treatment plan reflects significant changes in the individual's needs or current condition, including regression or progress.

Standard

TX.1.5.1 Rehabilitation services address assessed needs, in accordance with an individualized written plan of care developed by qualified and competent individuals.

Intent of TX.1.5.1

The information generated from assessment of the individual's physical, cognitive, communicative, emotional, and social status is integrated to identify the individual's rehabilitation needs. Rehabilitation services are initiated based on the individual's needs. Pharmacologic needs are assessed for individuals on long-term drug therapy. The treatment-planning process responds to those identified needs. The individual's written plan for rehabilitation guides delivery of services to meet identified needs.

Standard

TX.1.5.2 Justification is documented when identified needs are not addressed.

---

* **functional** Related to the actions and activities expected of a person.

Intent of TX.1.5.2

Treatment of certain needs may be appropriately addressed in continuing-care services after discharge. When those responsible for treatment planning and delivery decide not to address a need during the current period of treatment, they document their rationale in the clinical record.

Standard

TX.1.5.3 Individuals' perceptions of their needs are documented, as are the families' perceptions when appropriate and available.

Intent of TX.1.5.3

The organization documents the individual's expression of needs and priorities. When appropriate and available, family members participate in identifying what they consider to be the individual's needs, and their perceptions are documented as well. This documentation is available to those responsible for planning and providing treatment.

Standard

TX.1.5.4 Individuals are encouraged to participate in developing their treatment plans, and their involvement is documented.

Intent of TX.1.5.4

Individuals and care providers cooperate to achieve care goals. Care providers relate their clinical conclusions and treatment recommendations to each individual, and individuals are encouraged to participate in this process as much as they can. They are also encouraged to express their perceptions about whether specific concerns should be addressed. Ideally, as a participant in developing the treatment plan, the individual agrees with care providers about needs to be addressed and the time frame for addressing them.

All interventions respect individuals and their choices about participation in rehabilitation. Individuals are encouraged to make choices and develop a sense of achievement about progress.

Documentation of the nature and extent of individual involvement is often included in progress notes. It is not necessary for the individual to sign a specific treatment plan because a signature alone does not testify to the degree of involvement, understanding, or agreement in this important process.

Standards

TX.1.5.5 The treatment plan addresses the involvement of family when indicated.

TX.1.5.6 The treatment plan includes advocacy services when indicated to enhance the natural support system, facilitate environmental modifications, or create new supports.

Intent of TX.1.5.5 and TX.1.5.6

For many individuals, participation by family members will be a significant factor in achieving goals. The importance of participation by family in treatment planning is related to age or disability factors. Family members generally need to participate in the treatment of children and adolescents. Similarly, research indicates that family members' participation may facilitate treatment of alcohol and other drug problems and enhance the individual's potential for abstinence.

Family will also need to be actively involved when services are provided to severely and persistently mentally ill individuals and mentally retarded/developmentally disabled individuals who need continued training in activities of daily living (ADLs). In this case, significant others might include resident staff at a placement facility.

Generally, family participation may be documented in the treatment plan through problems or needs statements, goals, objectives, or the section of the treatment plan on interventions.

The expectations of advocates are considered and documented, as appropriate, in the rehabilitation plan. Also, the service provider is an advocate for the individual's needs and for improvements in the system, when needed.

Standards

TX.1.6 The treatment plan contains specific goals for achieving emotional and/or physical health as well as maximum growth and adaptive capabilities.

TX.1.6.1 Treatment-plan goals are based on assessments of the individual and, as appropriate, the family.

TX.1.6.2 Treatment-plan goals are linked to living, learning, and work activities.

Intent of TX.1.6 Through TX.1.6.2

Treatment goals are specific to problems and needs identified during the assessment process. Clearly defined problems and needs statements are necessary to establish such specific goals. In addition, treatment goals reflect individual and family expectations, as appropriate. Development of treatment goals will vary based on age or disability factors, and the goals may be narrowly focused, depending on anticipated length of stay or service.

A rehabilitation plan describes

- criteria for the transition to more independent and less restrictive environments and successful adaptation into natural or community settings; and
- the individual's skill and support requirements for living, learning, and work activities consistent with optimal independence and choice.

Consistent with individual goals, rehabilitation services help individuals meet skill and support requirements for living, learning, and work activities.

Standard

TX.1.7 The treatment plan includes specific objectives for the goals identified in the plan.

Intent of TX.1.7

For each identified treatment-planning goal, supporting objectives are developed. Objectives serve to operationalize individual treatment goals and form a framework guiding the provision of services. Objectives are expressed in behavioral terms that specify measurable indexes of progress. A time frame for achieving each objective is specified in the treatment plan.

Standard

TX.1.7.1 Rehabilitation plans include a description of facilitating factors and possible barriers to using rehabilitation services or reaching rehabilitation goals.

Intent of TX.1.7.1

The rehabilitation plan reflects the attainment of goals, successful role performance, changes in level of functioning, and efficiency of resource supports. The plan takes into account facilitating factors and barriers to reaching long-term rehabilitation goals. Barriers that might need to be considered include

- substance abuse and mental disorders;
- cognitive and communicative disorders;
- developmental disabilities;
- vision or hearing disabilities;
- physical disabilities;
- social and environmental.

Standard

TX.1.8 The treatment plan specifies the interventions and approaches necessary to meet the individual's needs and goals.

Intent of TX.1.8

The treatment plan specifies the services and interventions needed to meet the goals and objectives derived from assessing individual needs. The services and interventions specified may be described in further detail in program descriptions, such as a behavior management plan or therapy group protocol.

Standard

TX.1.8.1 When the individual's identified needs include developing skills for activities of daily living, a training program is developed.

Intent of TX.1.8.1

The training program specifies the program's behavioral objectives, the methods to be used, and the training schedule. Attention is given to the needs of individuals who, regardless of age or disability, may require training in activities of daily living (ADL), such as toileting, feeding, dressing, cooking, and cleaning. Activities of daily living may be a primary focus of the treatment plan for certain individuals, such as the mentally retarded/developmentally disabled (MR/DD). Individuals with severe or chronic disability or organic problems need to have more detailed treatment plans in this area, including specified objectives, methods, and training schedules. Children with autism or significant psychosis, adolescents in residential treatment, or individuals with severe and chronic psychiatric disorders may also require ADL training and treatment plan development.

Standard

TX.1.8.2 Activity services, when provided, are incorporated into the treatment plan to provide a consistent and well-structured framework.

Intent of TX.1.8.2

Activity services are specified in an individual's treatment plan. The scope and depth of the activities program are carefully matched with the individual's needs and balanced with free time and opportunity for additional therapeutic interaction with staff. Activity schedules are posted in locations accessible to both staff and individuals served.

Standard

TX.1.8.3 The treatment plan includes specialized rehabilitation services to restore or maintain the functional abilities of individuals with physical, cognitive, social, leisure, or sensoriperceptual impairments, or whose primary problem is mental illness.

Intent of TX.1.8.3

Individuals learn to apply skills gained during rehabilitation to their housing, vocational, educational, recreational, or social environments.

Standard

TX.1.8.4 When individuals need services not offered by the organization, appropriate referrals are made and documented in the clinical record.

Intent of TX.1.8.4

When needs are identified for which the organization does not directly provide services, the organization refers individuals to an outside source. These referrals are reflected in the clinical record. When concurrent services are an integral part of meeting the individual's needs, this documentation may be found in the treatment plan.

Standard

TX.1.9 The treatment plan specifies the frequency of treatment procedures.

Intent of TX.1.9

The frequency of treatment services, modalities, and procedures is identified to

- develop a specific treatment schedule for the individual; and
- provide a framework for charting progress notes in the clinical record.

Standard

TX.1.10 Goals are periodically evaluated and, when necessary, revised based on reassessment of the individual's current clinical problems, needs, and responses to treatment.

Intent of TX.1.10

This evaluation is conducted when major clinical changes occur and at specified regular intervals related to the individual's treatment. The treatment-planning process is designed to respond to individuals' current needs and clinical status over time, providing continuous, appropriate care. At regular intervals and in response to specific events, the plan is updated to reflect any changes in the individual's needs and responses to treatment.

Written policies and procedures specify the time frames and criteria for reviewing and updating treatment plans. During plan revision, problem statements, specific goals, treatment objectives, and treatment services are updated as necessary.

Standard

TX.1.11 The treatment plan stipulates specific criteria for discharge or terminating treatment.

Intent of TX.1.11

Discharge planning is initiated early in the treatment process based on requirements of the treatment plan or other written guidelines such as clinical pathways, including expected time frames for achieving goals and objectives. Criteria for discharge or terminating treatment may vary based on age and disability considerations and program objectives. Clinical criteria for individuals with chemical dependency problems will differ from those with psychiatric or emotional problems. Criteria for discharge will also vary by treatment setting in accordance with requirements of the organization's policies and procedures. (See also RI.1.1 and CC.6.1.1.)

Standards

TX.1.12 *In inpatient and residential programs, the organization's oral health program has mechanisms designed to meet individuals' oral health care needs. The objectives and scope of the oral health program include at least*

TX.1.12.1 in keeping with length of stay, the method(s) of providing, or referring individuals for, regular dental care;

TX.1.12.2 the method(s) of providing emergency dental care;

TX.1.12.3 daily oral hygiene procedures, including cleaning individuals' prostheses; and

TX.1.12.4 the proper labeling and storage of individuals' oral hygiene supplies and prostheses.

Intent of TX.1.12 Through TX.1.12.4

The objectives and scope of an oral health program are outlined in written policies and procedures. These policies and procedures identify the minimum length of stay for which an oral health program will be carried out. The organization establishes a means of providing or referring individuals for regular and emergency dental care. Daily oral hygiene procedures are also defined that, when appropriate, address cleaning individuals' prostheses (including appliances) as well as labeling and storing their oral hygiene supplies.

Treatment of Children and Adolescents

Standard

TX.1.13 Organization policy promotes access to appropriate educational services for each child or adolescent whose treatment causes a significant absence from school.

Intent of TX.1.13

It is important to maintain and, if possible, improve the academic achievement of children and adolescents who experience many absences from school while in treatment. A written policy addresses the role of education as a treatment activity and protects individuals from losing ground academically while in treatment. The organization defines the length of stay and absence from school that would require providing educational services.

Standard

TX.1.13.1 Educational services are designed to meet the child's or adolescent's treatment needs and to provide educational continuity.

Intent of TX.1.13.1

The organization facilitates educational continuity for children and adolescents in treatment by

- communicating with the individual's school regarding past academic functioning and achievement;
- promoting regular communication among teachers, clinical staff, and child care staff; and
- working to ensure consistent clinical intervention in both school and treatment, as defined in the treatment plan.

Program Plans for Individuals with Mental Retardation and Other Developmental Disabilities

Standard

TX.1.14 Programs offering services to individuals with mental retardation and other developmental disabilities accept and implement the independent living philosophy.*

Intent of TX.1.14

The independent living philosophy is incorporated into the organization's philosophy and carried forth in the services provided. To the extent feasible for each individual, the organization fosters a quality of life comparable to that experienced by most people.

The setting of services enhances and supports each individual's personal experiences, appearance, and behavior. The social and living environment offers a variety of social and community experiences facilitating the development of self-awareness, independence, and use of personal strengths and skills. Individuals participate in formulating policies that affect their living and social environment.

Standards

TX.1.15 A behavior management team develops an individualized program within 30 days of admission which it reviews and revises at key decision points, or at least annually.

TX.1.15.1 The plan is reviewed upon admission, transfer, and discharge and is revised as necessary.

TX.1.15.2 The plan is reviewed when major changes occur in presenting problems or disabilities and is revised as necessary.

---

* Independent living is the act or process of making available, to developmentally disabled individuals, patterns and conditions of everyday life that are as similar as possible to those of the mainstream of society, thereby enabling such individuals to enjoy a manner of living that is as close as possible to that considered normal in the community. The basic principle is that what is offered represents the least departure from normal patterns of living that can be effective in meeting the individuals' developmental needs.

TX.1.15.3 The plan is reviewed when introducing protective devices† or aversive consequences to address maladaptive behavior and is revised as necessary.

TX.1.15.4 The plan is reviewed when the individual reaches majority or emancipation and is revised as necessary.

TX.1.15.4.1 When individuals reach majority or emancipation, their civil and legal rights and, when appropriate, need for continued care or services are re-evaluated.

Intent of TX.1.15 Through TX.1.15.4.1

Timely development of an individualized plan for services is essential for mentally retarded/developmentally disabled individuals. Individualized program plans are reviewed and updated at least annually and according to individual needs. The organization establishes a list of criteria that trigger review of the program plan.

Standards

TX.1.16 Individuals or family members or advocates participate in individualized program planning, and their opinions and preferences about services, activities, and objectives are considered.

TX.1.16.1 Inability or unwillingness to participate in program planning is documented in the clinical record.

Intent of TX.1.16 and TX.1.16.1

Individuals and their families or advocates have the opportunity to participate in the planning process by expressing their opinions, preferences, questions, concerns, desires, and expectations for services. They should agree with the clinicians about needs to be addressed, methods to be used, and time frames established. Notes in the clinical record document their involvement or lack thereof.

Standards

TX.1.17 *When indicated to meet specified objectives, the clinical record addresses the use of corrective, adaptive, and prosthetic supports or devices and describes*

TX.1.17.1 the reason for their use; and

TX.1.17.2 how often and under what circumstances they will be used.

Intent of TX.1.17 Through TX.1.17.2

When corrective, adaptive, and prosthetic supports or devices are used, the clinical staff documents the following in individual program plans:

- the clinical condition that requires the supports or devices;
- the schedule or conditions for using the device or support; and
- the intended results of their use for the given individual in a clearly specified condition.

---

* See also Restraint and Seclusion standards, TX.3.1–TX.3.1.3.3.

Standards

TX.1.18 *When indicated to meet a specified objective, the clinical record addresses using training programs for activities of daily living (ADLs) and describes*

TX.1.18.1 the reason for such a program;

TX.1.18.2 how often and under what circumstances program activities will be conducted; and

TX.1.18.3 the methods to be used.

Intent of TX.1.18 Through TX.1.18.3

Clinical staff document the following in the clinical record:

- the individual needs to be addressed by training programs for ADLs;
- the schedule for the program's use or the situations in which program activities are initiated; and
- the intended results of such training when provided under clearly specified conditions.

Developing and recording this information will also produce criteria for evaluating the training program's effectiveness.

Standards

TX.1.19 *When indicated to meet a specified objective, the individual program plan addresses the use of behavior management procedures and describes*

TX.1.19.1 the reason for such procedures;

TX.1.19.2 the methods to be used;

TX.1.19.3 how often or under what circumstances they will be used; and

TX.1.19.4 any restriction of the individual's rights.

Intent of TX.1.19 Through TX.1.19.4

The clinical staff documents the following in the individual program plan:

- The problem behaviors that are the focus of behavior management procedures;
- The schedule for use or the specific circumstances in which they will be used;
- The intended result of behavior management procedures for the given individual when used in clearly specified conditions.

Developing and recording this information also produces criteria for measuring the effectiveness of behavior management programs against intended results.

Standard

TX.1.20 The organization provides for the health maintenance of all individuals served, including early detection and remediation of health needs.

Intent of TX.1.20

The organization is responsible for routinely monitoring each individual's physical health. Either directly or through referral to an outside source, the organization offers appropriate health services to address identified problems. The organization considers national preventive services guidelines for different segments of the population, such as those provided by the United States Preventive Services Task Force.

Standard

TX.1.20.1 Each individual's height is recorded in the clinical record.

Intent of TX.1.20.1

Height is monitored regularly as part of the health maintenance program. The frequency with which height is monitored is appropriate to the individual's age and growth potential. For a child or adolescent whose height may change rapidly over a period of time, height is recorded at least quarterly. For individuals who have reached the age of cessation of growth, height is recorded at least annually.

Standard

TX.1.20.2 When appropriate, an individual's weight is recorded in the clinical record at least quarterly.

Intent of TX.1.20.2

When appropriate, weight is monitored regularly as part of the individual's health maintenance program. Physicians or other qualified professionals participate in determining the criteria for including individuals in weight monitoring.

Standard

TX.1.20.3 The organization provides for corrective, adaptive, and prosthetic devices in accordance with assessment findings.

Intent of TX.1.20.3

The organization responds to physical limitations discovered during assessments with effective corrective action. Needed corrective, adaptive, or prosthetic devices are supplied either directly, through contractual arrangement, or by referral to an outside source.

Standard

TX.1.20.4 The organization implements written policies and procedures concerning detection of injury, disease, neglect, and abuse.

Intent of TX.1.20.4

The mentally retarded/developmentally disabled are at risk for unrecognized injury or disease. The organization establishes a written policy to help detect injury, disease, neglect, and abuse that the individual may not be able or willing to report. Procedures describe how these occurrences will be identified and clearly define typical signs of injury, disease, and abuse. These policies and procedures are incorporated in the staff development program.

Standard

TX.1.20.5 Seizure activity and periodic determination of anticonvulsant drug levels are accurately recorded in the individual's clinical record when indicated.

Intent of TX.1.20.5

Anticonvulsant drug levels are monitored regularly as part of the individual's health maintenance program, and the findings are documented in the clinical record. Physicians define the frequency and method of monitoring anticonvulsant drug levels.

Standard

TX.1.20.6 When physical therapy services are provided, they are supervised and coordinated by a qualified physical therapist.

Intent of TX.1.20.6

The organization is accountable for providing qualified staff to perform professional services, including physical therapy when provided. A qualified physical therapist is someone who is currently competent in the field, meets current legal requirements for licensure or registration, and either

- is a graduate of a physical therapy program approved by a nationally recognized accreditation body;
- meets any current legal requirements of licensure or registration; or
- has the documented equivalence in training, education, or experience.

Medication* Use

Medications are often an essential component of care and, when used, they require effective management. The following standards address four medication-use processes:

- prescription or ordering (TX.2.1–TX.2.1.2);
- preparation, dispensing, and storage (TX.2.2–TX.2.2.7);
- administration (TX.2.3–TX.2.3.3); and
- monitoring of effects (TX.2.4–TX.2.4.1).

Organizations surveyed under this manual identify which, if any, of these four processes they use. For example, if the organization observes the self-administration of medications and monitors their effects but does not prescribe, prepare, dispense, store, nor have staff administer medications, it would have to meet only the standards related to the self-administration of medications (TX.2.3.2) and the monitoring of their effects (TX.2.4–TX.2.4.1).

When pharmacologic agents are indicated for treating a diagnosed disorder, a physical assessment is conducted with respect to past and current drug treatments. The following issues are addressed for all past and current drug treatments:

- Efficacy;
- Impact on current and future functioning;

---

* **medication** Any substance, other than food or devices, intended for use in diagnosing, curing, mitigating, treating, or preventing disease.

- Side effects; and
- Evaluations of the drug treatments by the individual or family.

Pharmacologic interventions are coordinated with psychosocial interventions. Specific attention is given to side effects due to dosage levels or responses that interfere with an individual's ability to engage in psychosocial programming.

Standards

TX.2 *Systems and processes are implemented for the safe and effective use of medication.*

TX.2.1 The organization identifies an appropriate selection of medications available for prescription or ordering.*

TX.2.1.1 The organization establishes procedures for prescribing or ordering and procuring medications not available in the organization.

Intent of TX.2 Through TX.2.1.1

When the organization prescribes or orders and procures medications, it provides for their availability and safe and effective use. Appropriate staff collaboratively develop and maintain a list of medications available at all times for prescribing or ordering. These medications are selected on the basis of individual need and safety, not solely because of economics. Suggested criteria for selection include

- need in relation to the diseases and conditions treated by the organization;
- effectiveness, in terms of
  - efficacy (alone and in comparison to other products),
  - toxicity (alone and in comparison to other products),
  - pharmacokinetic properties,
  - bioequivalence† (if applicable),
  - pharmaceutical equivalence‡ (if applicable), and
  - therapeutic equivalence§ (if applicable); risks, including
  - known incidence of adverse drug reactions, and
  - potential for error in prescribing or ordering, preparing, dispensing, and administering; and
- acquisition costs and cost effects on the organization.

Standard

TX.2.1.2 Policies and procedures support safe prescription or ordering practices.

---

* **prescription or order** Directing the selection, preparation, and/or administration of medication(s).

† **bioequivalence** The degree to which two formulations of the same medication have equal bioavailability.[1]

[1] **bioavailability** The relative amount of and rate at which a medication dose reaches the systemic circulation in a therapeutically active form after administration.

‡ **pharmaceutical equivalence** The degree to which two formulations of the same medication are identical in strength, concentration, and dosage form.

§ **therapeutic equivalence** The degree to which two formulations of different active ingredients are judged by the clinical staff to have acceptably similar therapeutic effects.

Intent of TX.2.1.2

The organization develops and implements procedures that address

- ordering, procuring, storing, controlling, preparing, and dispensing medications according to law and regulation;
- distribution and administration of controlled medications, including adequate documentation and record keeping required by law;
- proper storage, distribution, and control of investigational medications and those in clinical trial;
- situations in which all or some of an individual's medication orders must be permanently or temporarily canceled, and mechanisms for reinstating them when appropriate;
- the qualification of "as needed" prescriptions or orders and times of dose administration;
- control of sample drugs;
- distribution of medications to individuals at home visits, therapeutic outings, and discharge;
- procurement, storage, control, and distribution of prepackaged medications obtained from an outside source when no on-site pharmacy service exists;
- if applicable, procurement, storage, control, distribution, and administration of radioactive medications;
- if applicable, procurement, storage, control, distribution, administration, and monitoring of blood derivatives*; and
- if applicable, procurement, storage, control, distribution, administration, and monitoring of radiographic contrast media.

Standard

TX.2.2 The preparation, dispensing, and storage of medications adhere to law, regulation, licensure, and professional standards of practice.

Intent of TX.2.2

When the organization prepares, dispenses, and stores medications, it demonstrates an understanding of, and compliance with, the applicable laws, regulations, professional licensure, and practice standards governing the provision of pharmacy services and use of medications.

Standards

TX.2.2.1 Medications are appropriately controlled during preparation and dispensing.

TX.2.2.2 If the organization prepares, dispenses, or stores medications, a medication-dose system is followed.

TX.2.2.3 A pharmacist reviews all prescriptions or orders.

Intent of TX.2.2.1 Through TX.2.2.3

Appropriate staff develop and maintain systems for controlling all medications stored at the organization, whether prepared by the organization's pharmacy service or obtained elsewhere by the individual. To ensure the safe and accurate dispensing of medications,

---

* **blood derivative** A pooled blood product, such as albumin, gamma globulin, or Rh immune globulin, whose use is considered significantly lower in risk than that of blood or blood components.

- a pharmacist reviews each prescription or order prior to dispensing (with the possible exceptions of emergency orders when time may not permit, and in situations in which a licensed independent practitioner with appropriate clinical privileges controls prescription, preparation, and administration);
- the pharmacist contacts the prescriber or orderer if questions arise;
- medications dispensed to both inpatients and outpatients are appropriately and safely labeled using a standardized method; and
- medications are dispensed in the most ready-to-administer form possible to minimize opportunities for error.

See also TX.2.2.5 which addresses providing medications when the pharmacy service is closed or access to medications is limited.

Standard

TX.2.2.4 Important individual medication information is captured, communicated, and considered when preparing and dispensing medications.

Intent of TX.2.2.4

To supplement monitoring of medication adverse events* and help ensure safe administration of medications, there is a system for informing the pharmacist and appropriate staff about the individual's medication regimen.

Standard

TX.2.2.5 Pharmacy services are available when the organization's pharmacy service is closed or not available or when access to medications is limited.

Intent of TX.2.2.5

Organizations that prepare, dispense, or store medications deliver consistent quality during all hours of service. To do this, they establish a means of providing pharmacy services when the pharmacy is closed, not available, or access to medications is otherwise limited.

Standard

TX.2.2.6 Emergency medication systems are available, when appropriate.

Intent of TX.2.2.6

The organization develops and maintains systems to ensure the availability, control, and security of emergency medications in the pharmacy service, as well as in treatment and care areas.

Standard

TX.2.2.7 A medication-recall system provides for retrieval and safe disposition of expired, and recalled medications.

* See the "Improving Organization Performance" chapter.

Intent of TX.2.2.7

The intent of this standard is self-evident. The prescribing physician is notified if an individual received a recalled or expired medication.

Standard

TX.2.3 Prescriptions or orders are verified and individuals are identified before medications are administered.

Intent of TX.2.3

To ensure safety and accuracy, when staff administer medications, they verify prescriptions or orders and the recipient's identity before administration. When administering medication, staff

- check to make sure the drug is stable and within expiration limits;
- verify that the drug is the correct drug ordered, in the prescribed strength, at the proper time and by the correct route of administration; and
- that the drug is not contraindicated for the patient.

Standard

TX.2.3.1 Qualified individuals administer medications.

Intent of TX.2.3.1

Staff members who administer medications are

- appropriately licensed or certified or trained when required by law and regulation; and
- knowledgeable about the medication they administer and the needs of the individual served.

Staff who administer medications receive training and appropriate information about:

- the nature of the medications to be administered;
- how to administer medications, e.g., the appropriate frequency, route, and dose;
- the expected actions and side effects of the medications to be administered; and
- how to monitor the effects of the medications on the individual.

Standard

TX.2.3.2 Systems are implemented to support self-administration or alternative medication administration systems.

Intent of TX.2.3.2

The organization safely manages medications brought into the organization by the individual. Self-administration of prescribed medications addresses drugs brought into the organization by an individual or those ordered by a licensed independent practitioner while the individual is in the organization. An individual's safe self-administration of medication is supported. Individuals permitted to self-administer medications do so only when specifically ordered by the responsible licensed independent practitioner. A clinical staff member supervises self-administration procedures.

Standard

TX.2.3.3 Investigational medications are safely controlled and administered.

Intent of TX.2.3.3

The organization protects the safety of individuals participating in investigational or clinical medication studies by ensuring that these activities are adequately controlled and supported.

Standards

TX.2.4 Medication's effect on the individual is monitored continuously.

TX.2.4.1 Effects of medication are assessed based on information maintained in the individual's clinical record and medication profile and observations by staff and the individual.

Intent of TX.2.4 and TX.2.4.1

Medication monitoring is a collaborative process that may include input from various disciplines and the individual and family, when appropriate. This information is used to maintain and improve the outcomes of drug therapy while minimizing any drug-related problems or adverse events.

Special Treatment Procedures

Certain clinical interventions are of particular interest from a risk-management standpoint. Clinicians using these interventions should ensure that their use is warranted and that individuals and their rights are always protected. Such treatment procedures include

- seclusion;
- restraint;
- electroconvulsive therapy and other forms of convulsive therapy;
- behavior-modification procedures that use painful stimuli;
- unusual medications and investigational and experimental drugs;
- maintenance use of drugs that have abuse potential, are known to involve a substantial risk, or are associated with undesirable side effects; and
- research projects that involve inconvenience or risk to the individual.

Standard

TX.3 *Designated special treatment procedures require clinical justification.*

Intent of TX.3

Special treatment procedures place individuals in a significantly more limited environment than the usual organizational setting. Because these interventions have the potential for neglect and abuse of the individual, health care providers document

- that such interventions are clinically justified;
- that less restrictive interventions were attempted first; and
- that the individual's condition was considered when using these interventions.

Restraint and Seclusion

Creating a physical, social, and cultural environment limiting restraint and seclusion use to clinically appropriate and adequately justified situations or that actually reduces their use through preventive or alternative strategies helps organization staff focus on the individual's well-being. The leaders' role is to help create such an environment. This requires planning and, frequently, new or reallocated resources, thoughtful education, and performance improvement. The result is an organization approach to restraint and seclusion that protects the individual's health and safety while preserving his or her dignity, rights, and well-being.

Restraint or seclusion may be used in response to emergent, dangerous behavior; addictive disorders; as an adjunct to planned care; as a component of an approved protocol; or, in some cases, as part of standard practice. Because restraint or seclusion may be necessary for certain individuals, health care organizations and providers need to be aware of the associated risks of both use and nonuse. They also need to be able to use restraint or seclusion when essential to protect individuals from harming themselves, other individuals, or staff.

In its broadest context, *restraint* is any method of physically restricting a person's freedom of movement, physical activity, or normal access to his or her body. In the context of these standards, restraint is considered involuntary use as either part of an approved protocol or as indicated by individual orders. *Seclusion* refers to the involuntary confinement of a person alone in a room where the person is physically prevented from leaving.

Restraint and seclusion have the potential to produce serious consequences, such as physical and psychological harm, loss of dignity, violation of an individual's rights, and even death. Due to the associated risks and consequences of use, organizations are increasingly exploring ways to decrease restraint and seclusion use through effective preventive strategies or the use of alternatives. For some organizations, a restraint- and seclusion-free environment is appropriate to their populations and clinical services, and can be achieved now or in the future. However, for many organizations, restraint or seclusion may continue to be necessary in clinically justified situations and in the foreseeable future, given the organization's populations and clinical services, the current state of knowledge, and available effective alternatives.

These standards for restraint and seclusion address processes and activities that

- identify areas of organization leadership and action that will limit restraint and seclusion use to clinically justified situations and may, when appropriate, seek to reduce restraint use through performance improvement;
- guide an organization's efforts to prevent the need to restrain or seclude individuals; and
- provide a framework focused on the individual to guide any actual restraint or seclusion use through clinical protocols or individual orders.

Standard(s)

- TX.3.1.1 through TX.3.1.1.7 address limiting restraint and seclusion;
- TX.3.1.2 addresses reducing restraint and seclusion as part of performance improvement;
- TX.3.1.3 addresses the policies and procedures associated with restraint and seclusion;
- TX.3.1.3.1 through TX.3.1.3.1.3 address restraint and seclusion as a component of an approved clinical protocol;
- TX.3.1.3.2 through TX.3.1.3.2.8 address restraint and seclusion initiated through individual orders; and
- TX.3.1.3.3 addresses clinical record documentation.

Note: *Standards TX.3.1 through TX.3.1.3.3 apply to any organization where restraint or seclusion is initiated by individual orders or approved protocols of care.*

The standards do not apply to restraint associated only with medical, dental, diagnostic, or surgical procedures and are based on standard practice for the procedure. Such standard practice may or may not be described in procedure or practice descriptions. For example, the standards do not apply to medical immobilization in the form of surgical positioning, IV arm boards, radiotherapy procedures, electroconvulsive therapy, and so on.

The standards do not apply when a restraint device is used to meet the assessed needs of an individual who requires adaptive support (for example, postural support, orthopedic appliances) or medical protective devices (for example, helmets, tabletop chairs, bed rails). Such use is always based on the assessed needs of the individual. Periodic reassessment ensures that the restraint continues to meet an identified individual need.

The standards do not apply to therapeutic holding or comforting of children or to a time-out when the person to whom it is applied is physically prevented from leaving a room for 15 minutes or less and when its use is consistent with the behavior management standards.

The standards do not apply to forensic and correction restrictions used for security purposes. However, restraint or seclusion use related to the clinical care of an individual under forensic or correction restrictions is surveyed under these standards.

Standard

TX.3.1 Restraint or seclusion use within the organization is limited to those situations with adequate, appropriate clinical justification.

Intent of TX.3.1

Limiting the use of restraint or seclusion to clinically justified situations requires clear policies and procedures, well-trained staff, and the support of the organization's leaders and culture.

Clinical justification can be guided by clear criteria in practice guidelines, practice parameters, pathways of care, or other standardized care processes from relevant professional organizations. When not available, the qualified staff of an organization establishes criteria or otherwise guides justification for the population served and clinical services provided by the organization.

Standards

TX.3.1.1 *Organization leaders support limited, justified use of restraint or seclusion through the following:*

TX.3.1.1.1 Plans, policies, and priorities;

TX.3.1.1.2 *Human resource planning;*

TX.3.1.1.3 *Staff orientation and education that creates a culture emphasizing prevention and appropriate use and encouraging alternatives;*

TX.3.1.1.4 Education of the individual and, when appropriate, his or her family;

TX.3.1.1.5 Assessment processes that identify and, when appropriate, prevent potential behavioral risk factors;

TX.3.1.1.6 Design and delivery of care; and

TX.3.1.1.7 The development and promotion of preventive strategies and use of safe and effective alternatives.

Intent of TX.3.1.1 Through TX.3.1.1.7

Limiting the use of restraint or seclusion to those situations with appropriate and adequate clinical justification requires

- effective leadership to shape the culture of the organization;
- supportive plans, policies, and priorities;
- an understanding of the human-resource implications of limited use and choices related to reduced use;
- ongoing staff orientation and education;
- education of the individual and, when appropriate, his or her family; and
- the integration of restraint and seclusion into the organization's performance improvement activities.

In particular, attention is directed toward

- refining behavioral health, medical, dental, surgical, and diagnostic assessment processes to identify earlier the potential risk of dangerous behavior and the prevention, when appropriate, of those behaviors;
- reviewing and, when necessary, redesigning care processes associated with restraint and seclusion use; and
- identifying, developing, and promoting preventive strategies and the use of safe and effective alternatives.

Standard

TX.3.1.2 Performance improvement processes identify opportunities, when appropriate, to reduce restraint or seclusion use.

Intent of TX.3.1.2

Restraint and seclusion are high risk and problem prone. Thus they are a logical component of an organization's performance improvement program. The measurement and assessment process for restraint and seclusion seeks to understand the root cause of their use and incorporates this understanding into the organization's plans and priorities to evaluate and, if appropriate, reduce their use. This understanding is advanced by assessing aggregate data on restraint and seclusion episodes from all units, for all shifts, and for all purposes for which restraint and seclusion are used. Particular attention is paid to instances of multiple episodes of use for one individual and the frequency of restraint use by type(s) of staff.

Standard

TX.3.1.3 When restraint or seclusion is used, organization policy and procedures guide appropriate and safe use.

Intent of TX.3.1.3

Several essential elements govern how an organization uses restraint and seclusion appropriately for the population and individuals served. These elements focus on the individual and are described in organization policy(ies) and procedure(s) and include appropriate details as to how the organization

- protects and preserves the individual's rights, dignity, and well-being during use;
- bases use on the individual's assessed needs;
- makes decisions about least restrictive methods;
- ensures safe application and removal by competent staff;
- monitors and reassesses the individual during use;
- provides for the individual's needs during use;
- limits individual orders to licensed independent practitioners;
- time-limits orders; and
- documents in the clinical record when restraint or seclusion clinical protocols are used or individual orders written.

These essential elements help ensure that any use of restraint or seclusion, even when initiated by a protocol, protects and preserves the individual and his or her rights, dignity, and well-being. Appropriate staff approve policies and procedures for restraint and seclusion.

Standards

TX.3.1.3.1 Protocols that guide using restraint as an integral component of medical, dental, diagnostic, or surgical procedures or devices are consistent with organization policy.

TX.3.1.3.1.1 The appropriate clinical staff approve the protocols.

TX.3.1.3.1.2 Criteria are used to select individuals for care under the protocol.

TX.3.1.3.1.3 Qualified staff are identified and permitted to apply the criteria.

Intent of TX.3.1.3.1 Through TX.3.1.3.1.3

Restraint use guided by a clinical care protocol is consistent with written policies for restraint as described in the intent of TX.3.1.3. Such protocols are based on professional practice standards and focus on the individual, reducing health and safety risks and protecting the individual's rights and dignity. The appropriate clinical staff approve the protocol.

Restraint use guided by a protocol is initiated and terminated by qualified staff through the application of criteria.

Standard

TX.3.1.3.2 *Individual orders for restraint or seclusion are consistent with organization policy.*

Intent of TX.3.1.3.2

Individual orders are the most common source for initiating restraint or seclusion, especially in behavioral health settings. Who is authorized to order restraint or seclusion, how orders are conveyed, the details given in an order (for example, those related to time limits), and who is authorized to carry out the order are all essential aspects of processes to protect the individual served, other individuals, and staff.

Standard

TX.3.1.3.2.1 Individuals' rights, dignity, and well-being are protected during restraint or seclusion use.

Intent of TX.3.1.3.2.1

Each individual has the right to respectful care that maintains his or her dignity. Restraint and seclusion have the potential to significantly restrict these rights and can have serious adverse effects on the individual's well-being. Thus, each episode of use considers how the intervention will affect the individual, including whether

- the application or initiation respects the individual;
- the environment is safe and clean;
- the individual is able to continue his or her care and participate in care processes; and
- modesty, visibility to others, and comfortable body temperature are maintained.

Standard

TX.3.1.3.2.2 Restraint or seclusion use is based on the assessed needs of the individual.

Intent of TX.3.1.3.2.2

Single episodes of use or continued use of restraint or seclusion is based on the individual's needs, as identified in the initial assessment process or by qualified staff in emergent situations that pose the risk of injury to self or others. Therefore, there is clinical justification for each episode of use, including emergency use when a licensed independent practitioner is not available.

Use is not based solely on previous history of use or history of dangerous behavior. Rather, use is based on the individual's needs in the immediate care environment and the interaction of the individual with staff and other individuals in that environment. The organization does not permit any other use, such as for punishment or staff convenience.

Use appropriate to the needs of the individual is ensured by

- the training and skill of those who decide to apply restraint or initiate seclusion for emergency reasons in the absence of a licensed independent practitioner;
- clinical oversight by a licensed independent practitioner;
- review and evaluation of multiple episodes of use or continuous use; and
- organization policy.

Standard

TX.3.1.3.2.3 The least restrictive, safe, and effective restraint or seclusion method is used.

Intent of TX.3.1.3.2.3

The choice of restraint or seclusion method is guided by policy. The choice of the least restrictive, safe, and effective method for an individual is determined by the individual's assessed needs and the effective or ineffective methods previously used on the individual. In the absence of previous experience, policy describes typical circumstances under which the least restrictive methods should be tried first and explains how to use the methods. Once used, monitoring and reassessment of the individual ensures that less restrictive methods are used when possible and use is discontinued as soon as possible. The safety of both the individual and staff are considered in making these decisions.

Standard

TX.3.1.3.2.4 Restraint or seclusion is used correctly by competent, trained staff.

Intent of TX.3.1.3.2.4

Competent staff are essential to using restraint or seclusion safely and effectively and to protecting the individual during use. Appropriate use of restraint or seclusion is necessary if the individual's rights are to be respected and harm to the individual avoided. The organization identifies, educates, and determines the competency of those staff members who apply or remove restraint or who initiate or terminate seclusion. Frequently repeated in-service education, including an understanding of manufacturer's instructions for use of restraint devices, helps ensure safe use.

If possible, and as appropriate to the population and methods used, the insights of individuals who have experienced being placed in restraints are included to help staff better understand all aspects of their use.

Standard

TX.3.1.3.2.5 Individuals in restraint or seclusion are monitored and reassessed appropriately.

Intent of TX.3.1.3.2.5

Individuals can experience harm, unintentional limitation of their rights and dignity, deterioration in well-being, and feelings of isolation when restraint or seclusion methods are used. Monitoring is essential to prevent or reduce such occurrences. Reassessment during monitoring permits the reduction or early termination of restraint or seclusion.

Organization policy defines the nature and extent of appropriate monitoring by observation and direct, face-to-face interaction with the individual, and defines the monitoring frequency as continuous or no less frequent than every 15 minutes.

Reassessment associated with monitoring is used primarily to determine the individual's well-being, and reassessment of time-limited orders is used mainly to determine the continuing need for restraint or seclusion.

Standard

TX.3.1.3.2.6 The needs of the individual are met during restraint or seclusion use.

Intent of TX.3.1.3.2.6

The individual's physical and emotional needs are considered while the individual is in restraint or seclusion. The basic rights of human dignity and respect are maintained, and physical well-being is preserved through adequate exercise, nourishment, and personal care.

Standard

TX.3.1.3.2.7 Restraint or seclusion use is ordered by a licensed independent practitioner*.

Intent of TX.3.1.3.2.7

Licensed independent practitioners oversee how the assessed needs of individuals they are responsible for are met. This requires knowledge about and involvement in any use of restraint and seclusion.

---

* **licensed independent practitioner** Any individual who is permitted by law and who is also permitted by the organization to provide care services without direction or supervision, within the scope of his or her license, and in accordance with individually granted clinical privileges.

Each licensed independent practitioner can best carry out his or her responsibility when he or she

- provides verbal or written orders for initial use or to reauthorize continuing emergency use;
- participates in daily reviews of restraint and seclusion use for the individuals in his or her care; and
- participates in measuring and assessing use for all individuals within the organization.

Organization policy identifies who (in accordance with state law) is authorized by the organization to give verbal or written orders for restraint or seclusion and who may receive, record, and initiate verbal orders. Organization policy also identifies the process for reviewing and reauthorizing emergency restraint or seclusion use.

The organization may authorize an individual who is not a licensed independent practitioner to order emergency restraint or seclusion use in response to an individual who poses an immediate danger to himself or herself or to others. When such emergency use is initiated, a licensed independent practitioner is called within one hour. Continued use depends on authorization by a licensed independent practitioner.

Standard

TX.3.1.3.2.8 Orders for restraint or seclusion define specific time limits.

Intent of TX.3.1.3.2.8

Time-limited orders. Written orders for restraint and seclusion are limited to

- 4 hours for adults;
- 2 hours for children and adolescents ages 9 to 17; or
- 1 hour for children under age 9.

Early release. Staff can use criteria to guide early restraint or seclusion termination. When restraint or seclusion is terminated early and the same behavior is still evident, the original order can be reapplied if alternatives remain ineffective.

Continuation of orders. After the original order expires, the individual receives a face-to-face reassessment by a licensed independent practitioner. The licensed independent practitioner writes a new order if restraint or seclusion is to be continued. Organization policy and the original order may permit a licensed, qualified, and authorized individual (such as a registered nurse) to perform the reassessment and make a decision to continue the original order for an additional

- 4 hours for adults up to a maximum of 24 hours;
- 2 hours for children and adolescents ages 9 to 17 up to a maximum of 24 hours; or
- 1 hour for children under age 9 for periods up to a maximum of 24 hours.

Continuation of orders cannot under any circumstances exceed 24 hours without a face-to-face reassessment by a licensed independent practitioner and a new order.

PRN orders. PRN orders, whether individual or as part of a protocol, are prohibited.

Standard

TX.3.1.3.3 Documentation in clinical records reflects organization policy.

Intent of TX.3.1.3.3

The use of restraint or seclusion is recorded in the individual's clinical record. The purpose and focus of an entry(ies) is on the individual.

Each episode of use is recorded and includes

- clinical justification for use;

- orders for restraint or seclusion that meet the requirements described in organization policy; and
- measures taken to protect the rights, dignity, and well-being of the individual including monitoring, reassessment, and attention to needs.

Other Special Procedures

Standard

TX.3.2 Policies and procedures govern the use of electroconvulsive therapy and other forms of convulsive therapy.

Intent of TX.3.2

The governing body, administration, and clinical staff establish policies and consistent processes to control the use of these special and high-risk interventions.

Before initiating electroconvulsive therapy for a child or adolescent, two qualified child psychiatrists must concur with the treatment. These psychiatrists must be trained or experienced in treating children and adolescents and not directly involved in treating the individual. Both must

- examine the individual;
- consult with the responsible psychiatrist; and
- document their concurrence with the treatment in the individual's record.

Standard

TX.3.2.1 Written consent for any use of electroconvulsive therapy or other forms of convulsive therapy is obtained from the individual and documented in the clinical record.

Intent of TX.3.2.1

Because convulsive therapies raise societal and individual rights concerns, fully documented and fully informed consent is essential to protect individuals served, staff, and the organization. Steps are taken and documented to ensure that consent is fully informed and based on enough information to enable valid decision making by the individual or family. Individuals giving consent must be legally authorized and competent to do so, and provisions are made for withdrawal of consent.

These interventions are of particular concern when used to treat children and adolescents. Therefore, careful and detailed documentation is required in these instances.

Standard

TX.3.3 Policies and procedures govern the use of unusual medications and investigational and experimental drugs.

Intent of TX.3.3

Special risk-management concerns are raised by medications that carry an unusually high risk of side effects or undesirable reactions or for which clinical safety and efficacy have not been fully established. Current, comprehensive, written policies and procedures guide the use of such medications. Monitoring helps ensure adherence to all requirements of these policies and procedures.

Standard

TX.3.3.1 Investigational drugs are used only under the principal investigator's supervision and with the approval of the physician members of the clinical staff or an appropriate clinical staff committee, the research review committee, and appropriate federal, state, and local agencies.

Intent of TX.3.3.1

Recognizing sensitivity to the use of particular populations for experimentation and research, the organization uses a well-documented process of approval, supervision, and monitoring when using investigational drugs.

Standard

TX.3.4 Policies and procedures govern maintenance use of drugs that have abuse potential (usually considered to be controlled substances and drugs which can be used as chemical restraints), are known to involve substantial risk, or are associated with significant, undesirable side effects.

Intent of TX.3.4

Clear direction and control in drug prescription and administration are instituted to allay public and professional concerns about the side effects of medications, adverse reactions to medications, and misuse of prescribing authority (misuse of prescribing drugs with abuse potential). If psychopharmacologic drugs are used, the organization's governing body, administration, and clinical staff establish written policies and procedures addressing

- multiple psychopharmacologic agents;
- high-dose pharmacotherapy; and
- prevention, identification, and management of tardive dyskinesia.

Standard

TX.3.4.1 The organization's list of selected medications includes prescribed and administered maintenance drugs that have abuse potential.

Intent of TX.3.4.1

A physician documents in the individual's clinical record both the need and rationale for prescribing and administering maintenance drugs with abuse potential. Such drugs have been identified as an appropriate selection of medications available for prescription or ordering as part of the list described in TX.3.1.

Behavior Management

Standard

TX.3.5 Policies and procedures govern the use of behavior management procedures for controlling maladaptive or problem behavior.

Intent of TX.3.5

The clinical leaders establish a clear, comprehensive framework for using behavior management procedures.

Standards

TX.3.5.1 The organization requires a positive approach to behavior management and the progressive use of the least restrictive alternatives.

TX.3.5.2 The clinical leaders specify and approve the behavior management procedures that can be used in the organization.

TX.3.5.3 Behavior management programs identify and teach the individual appropriate expression of the target behavior or alternative adaptive behaviors.

TX.3.5.4 Procedures that may result in denying a nutritionally adequate diet are prohibited.

TX.3.5.5 Seclusion other than in accordance with standards in this chapter is prohibited.

TX.3.5.6 Corporal punishment is prohibited.

TX.3.5.7 Fear-eliciting procedures are prohibited.

TX.3.5.8 Other individuals served by the organization's services are prohibited from carrying out an individual's behavior management program.

Intent of TX.3.5.1 Through TX.3.5.8

Behavior management programs represent an important clinical intervention to address maladaptive or problem behaviors. However, these programs also present a potential for physical as well as psychological risk when used without adequate care. Least restrictive methods are always tried first, and if ineffective, only then are progressively more restrictive methods used. Policy specifies the aspects of behavior management programs that clinical leaders should consider when reviewing individual behavior management programs.

Standard

TX.3.5.9 A behavior management committee established by the clinical staff reviews, evaluates, and approves all behavior management programs.

Intent of TX.3.5.9

Consistent with its responsibility for promoting the quality of care, the organization leaders identify behavior management as a clinical activity that warrants careful review and evaluation. A behavior management committee performs the review and evaluation, and ensures that behavior management programs are initiated only with its approval.

Standard

TX.3.5.10 Time-out is used in accordance with the individual's program plan and the organization's policies and procedures.

Intent of TX.3.5.10

Time-out is identified as a clinical intervention. As such, it is used only when specific need for it and has defined objectives and conditions for its use in the individual program plan.

Well-defined, written policies and procedures provide a clear framework for using time-outs. The organization's leaders may delegate responsibility for developing written time-out policies and procedures to the behavior management committee.

Standard

TX.3.5.11 Aversive behavioral consequences are used only when withholding this intervention would be contrary to the individual's best interests and less restrictive alternatives have failed.

Intent of TX.3.5.11

When behavior management programs call for using aversive behavioral consequences, there is clear documentation in the clinical record that the program's target behavior is seriously detrimental to the individual's physical health or is a significant obstacle to normalization. Documentation of the failure of positive-reinforcement techniques is also documented in the clinical record before aversive behavioral consequences are used.

Standard

TX.3.5.12 Aversive behavioral consequences for maladaptive behavior are used in accordance with the individual's behavior management plan and organization policies and procedures.

Intent of TX.3.5.12

Using aversive behavioral consequences as clinical interventions is appropriate only when the interdisciplinary team has identified a need and defined objectives and conditions for its use in the individual behavior management plan. Well-defined, written policies and procedures provide a clear framework for using aversive behavioral consequences. The clinical staff may delegate responsibility for developing these policies and procedures to the behavior management committee.

Treatment in Forensic Services

Standards

TX.3.6 *Legal, correctional, and/or administrative decisions affecting an individual's treatment are coordinated with clinical decisions, including those related to*

TX.3.6.1 use of seclusion and restraint for nonclinical purposes;

TX.3.6.2 imposition of disciplinary restrictions;

TX.3.6.3 length of stay;

TX.3.6.4 restriction of rights; and

TX.3.6.5 plan for discharge and continuing care.

Intent of TX.3.6 Through TX.3.6.5

Nonclinical constraints affect admission, treatment, and discharge decisions in organizations providing forensic services. Such an organization often must accept court-ordered admission and has limited ability to select the type of individuals it will serve. In addition, such organizations often cannot limit their admissions to individuals requiring the level of care and services they offer. That is, such organizations are also required by the courts and the forensic system to admit, to 24-hour care, a significant number of individuals who may not require mental health services or who could be adequately served on an outpatient or partial-hospitalization basis if security were not a concern. Furthermore, such an organization often cannot give individuals increasing freedom (for example, community visits) as part of their treatment program or discharge them without a court order. Therefore, the facility coordinates its clinical decisions with these constraints when applicable.

Nutrition Care*

For the majority of behavioral health care providers, nutrition assessment, care planning, and service delivery are evaluated for compliance with standards found in the chapter on "Assessment" and standards TX.1 through TX.1.11 in this chapter on "Care."

When screening assessments find that an individual is at moderate or high risk of nutrition problems, the organization is not required to provide the in-depth nutrition assessments or care and treatment. The organization is expected to refer the individual to another organization or qualified professional who can assess and manage the level of nutrition care required by the individual consistent with the requirements found in the "Continuum" chapter.

When a behavioral health care organization does provide nutritional assessments or care and treatment of nutritional problems (including providing enteral products), the following standards apply in addition to those noted above for assessment, reassessments, care planning, and provision of care:

- Rights, Responsibilities, and Ethics;
- Continuum;
- Assessment;
- Education;

---

* **nutrition care** Interventions and counseling of individuals on appropriate nutrition[1] intake by integrating information from a nutrition assessment[2] with information on food and other sources of nutrients and meal preparation consistent with cultural background and socioeconomic status. Nutrition therapy, a component of medical treatment, includes enteral[3] and parenteral nutrition.[4]

[1] **nutrition** The sum of the processes by which one takes in and uses nutrients (protein, carbohydrate, lipids, vitamins, electrolytes, minerals, and water).

[2] **nutrition assessment** The comprehensive approach to defining nutrition status, which employs medical, nutrition, and medication intake histories; physical examination; anthropometric measurements; and laboratory data.

[3] **enteral nutrition** Nutrition provided via the gastrointestinal tract. Enteral nutrition encompasses both oral (delivered through the mouth) or tube (provided through a tube or catheter that delivers nutrients distal to the mouth) routes.

[4] **parenteral nutrition** Appropriate nutrition for those individuals who have lost gastrointestinal function or who cannot maintain adequate nutrition care status through conventional intake of nutrients. Through parenteral nutrition, all daily nutrition requirements to effect protein synthesis and maintain adequate nutrition status can be safely administered through a variety of veins.

- Improving Organization Performance; and
- Management of Human Resources.

These standards focus on providing appropriate nutrition care, including food and nutrition therapy, in a timely, effective, and efficient manner using all appropriate resources.

Like all individual care, nutrition care is an interdisciplinary process. Nutrition care teams may include physicians, registered dietitians,* nurses, pharmacists, and members of other disciplines as appropriate.

Nutrition care consists of the following processes:

- Screening, assessing, and reassessing nutrition needs;
- Developing the plan for nutrition therapy;
- Prescribing or ordering food and other nutrients;
- Preparing and distributing or administering food and other nutrients; and
- Monitoring the response of the individual served to nutrition care.

Standard

TX.4 The plan for nutrition care is developed and, when necessary, revised through a process whenever appropriate to the individual served.

Intent of TX.4

A nutrition care plan is developed for all individuals based on the results of the nutrition screen, the nutrition assessment and reassessment (as appropriate), and the individual's cultural, ethnic, and personal needs and preferences.

Standard

TX.4.1 Authorized individuals prescribe or order nutrition care in a timely manner.

Intent of TX.4.1

Food and nutrition therapies are administered to individuals only upon the order of appropriately authorized individuals.

Standard

TX.4.2 The organization defines and assigns responsibility for preparing, storing, distributing, and administering food and nutrition therapy products.

Intent of TX.4.2

To provide safe and accurate food and nutrition therapy, the responsibility for preparation, storage, distribution, and administration activities is clearly defined and assigned. These activities may be assigned to members of various disciplines within the organization.

Nutrition care prescriptions or orders are communicated in a timely and accurate manner to the individuals responsible for preparation, such as the nutrition care or pharmacy service. The

---

* **registered dietitian** The Commission on Dietetic Registration, the credentialing agent of the American Dietetic Association, defines the registered dietitian as an individual who 1) completed the minimum of a baccalaureate degree granted by a U.S. regionally accredited college or university; 2) met current academic requirements (Didactic Program in Dietetics) as approved by the American Dietetic Association; 3) completed preprofessional experience accredited or approved by the American Dietetic Association; 4) successfully completed the Registration Examination for Dietitians; and 5) accrued 78 hours of approved continuing education every five years.

organization defines what constitutes timely communication and establishes a method of determining accuracy of prescriptions or orders received. Prescriptions or orders are verified with the prescriber or orderer if there is a question or discrepancy.

Standard

TX.4.3 Food and nutrition therapy products are distributed and administered in a safe, accurate, and timely manner to the individual for whom they were prescribed or ordered.

Intent of TX.4.3

Food and nutrition therapy products, including parenteral nutrition, are distributed and administered to individuals in a safe, accurate, efficient, and, in the case of food, appetizing manner.

Standard

TX.4.4 The organization has a process for providing food or nutrition therapy when diets or diet schedules are altered.

Intent of TX.4.4

Accountability must be defined to effectively provide food or nutrition therapy to individuals who do not receive the regular meal service. The nutrition distribution and administration system can accommodate the unique needs of individuals who are not subject to the routine food or nutrition therapy delivery schedule or services. The needs of individuals not receiving the regular meal service or whose food or nutrition therapy comes from a source outside the institution, for example, are also identified and effectively accommodated.

Standard

TX.4.5 Each individual is monitored for the nutrition's effectiveness and appropriateness.

Intent of TX.4.5

Ongoing nutrition-care monitoring is essential to ensure effectiveness, appropriateness, and continuity of care. Members of the clinical team share responsibility for this process.

This standard is not intended to add documentation to existing forms or methods of monitoring. It should, however, focus the clinical team on the results of the collaborative effort of nutritional care monitoring.

Standard

TX.4.6 Nutrition care approaches and processes are standardized and communicated throughout the organization.

Intent of TX.4.6

Appropriate staff collaboratively develop a system for ensuring consistent standards in food and nutrition therapy. Standardized approaches and practices are communicated throughout the organization.

Physical Therapy Care and Services

Standard

TX.5 An initial physical therapy evaluation and assessment are conducted before physical therapy services are provided.

Intent of TX.5

The individual's physical status and functional abilities are evaluated before instruction and treatments are initiated.

Standard

TX.5.1 Whenever physical therapy is provided, treatment goals and plans are developed that are consistent with the diagnosis, the prognosis, and the aim of preventing or reducing disability or pain and restoring lost function.

Intent of TX.5.1

Physical therapy goals and plans are designed to help individuals achieve and maintain their optimal level of functioning, self-care, and independence by

- managing the individual's specific health problems; and
- maximizing the individual's emotional well-being in accordance with the diagnosis, prognosis, and treatment program.

Standard

TX.5.2 Whenever physical therapy is provided, planned services include therapeutic interventions that enhance daily living.

Intent of TX.5.2

Physical limitations discovered during the rehabilitation assessment are addressed with therapeutic interventions that enhance functional daily living skills and abilities. The plan reflects the clinical conditions requiring the use, application, and intended results of modalities, therapeutic exercises, and orthotic, prosthetic, and assistive devices. These interventions address posture, locomotion, strength, endurance, cardiopulmonary function, balance, coordination, joint mobility, flexibility, and pain. Applied modalities include, but are not limited to, heat, cold, light, air, water, sound, electricity, massage, mobilization, and bronchopulmonary hygiene. These interventions are provided either directly or through referrals, outside sources, or other arrangements.

Standard

TX.5.3 Physical therapy staff monitor the extent to which services have met the therapeutic goals established through assessments, caused improvement of the identified physical dysfunction, or reduced pain associated with movement.

Intent of TX.5.3

Staff periodically assess physical rehabilitation achievement and potential for each individual. Periodic reassessments are performed, as needed, to review treatment goals. (See also PE.3–PE.3.3.)

Anesthesia* Care

Introduction

The standards for anesthesia care apply when individuals served in any setting, for any purpose, and by any route receive

1. general, spinal, or other major regional anesthesia; or
2. sedation (with or without analgesia) that, in the manner used, may be reasonably expected to result in the loss of protective reflexes.

Because sedation is a continuum, it is not always possible to predict how an individual receiving sedation will respond. Therefore, each organization develops specific, appropriate protocols for the care of individuals receiving sedation that carries the risk of loss of protective reflexes†. These protocols are consistent with professional standards and address

- the presence of enough qualified individuals on staff‡ to perform the procedure and monitor the individual served;§
- appropriate equipment for care and resuscitation;**
- appropriate monitoring of vital signs—heart and respiratory rates and oxygenation using pulse oximetry equipment;††
- documentation of care,‡‡ and
- monitoring of outcomes.§§

Standard

TX.6 *A preanesthesia assessment is completed before anesthesia is administered.*

Intent of TX.6

A preanesthesia assessment is conducted whenever anesthesia is to be administered. The purpose of this assessment is to collect information needed to

- plan the choice of anesthesia care for the individual;
- safely administer anesthesia; and
- interpret findings while monitoring the individual.

---

* **anesthesia** The administration (in any surveyed setting, by any route, for any purpose) of general, spinal, or other major regional anesthesia or sedation with or without analgesia for which there is a reasonable expectation that, in the manner used, the sedation or analgesia will result in the loss of protective reflexes for a significant percentage of a group of individuals.

† **loss of protective reflexes** An inability to handle secretions without aspiration or to maintain a patent airway independently.

‡ **qualified individual** An individual who is qualified to participate in one or all of the mechanism outlined in the standards by virtue of one or more of the following: education, experience, competence, applicable professional licensure, regulation, and/or certification, registration, and privileges.

§ See TX.6 through TX.6.4.1.1.

** See standards LD.2.9 and EC.2.8.2.

†† See TX.6 through TX.6.4.1.1.

‡‡ See IM.7.4 through IM.7.4.3.6.

§§ See LD.4.3 and PI.3.1.

Standard

TX.6.1 A plan for anesthesia care is developed.

Intent of TX.6.1

Each individual's anesthesia care is planned to ensure that individual needs are met and safety is protected.

Standard

TX.6.2 Anesthesia options and risks are addressed with the individual and family, if appropriate.

Intent of TX.6.2

Given enough information, individuals and families can participate in care decisions. Before consent is obtained, risks, benefits, and alternatives to the planned procedure(s) are discussed.

Standard

TX.6.3 The individual's physiological and neurological status is measured and assessed during the administration of anesthesia.

Intent of TX.6.3

The organization ensures that all individuals are appropriately monitored during the administration of anesthesia and while under anesthesia. Physiological monitoring is the only reliable source of assessment information for individuals who have lost consciousness or protective reflexes, such as an inability to handle secretions without aspiration or to maintain a patent airway independently. Monitoring methods depend on the individual's preprocedure status and the choice of anesthesia.

Standards

TX.6.4 *The individual's postprocedure status is assessed on admission to and before discharge from the postanesthesia recovery area or the setting.*

TX.6.4.1 Individuals are discharged from the recovery area by a qualified licensed independent practitioner* or according to approved criteria.

TX.6.4.1.1 *When discharge criteria are used, compliance with the criteria is fully documented in the individual's clinical record.*

Intent of TX.6.4 Through TX.6.4.1.1

To ensure safe postprocedure and postanesthesia care, individuals are reassessed on a continuing basis and at critical transitions by qualified staff. Individuals are discharged from the postanesthesia recovery area either by licensed independent practitioners or according to approved criteria. The criteria are approved by the licensed physicians of the clinical staff and are rigorously applied to determine the individual's readiness for discharge.

---

* **licensed independent practitioner** Any individual permitted by law and by the organization to provide care services without direction or supervision, within the scope of the individual's licensure or certification and in accordance with individually granted clinical privileges (these individuals may also be referred to by other terms such as "independent care provider").

Education

Overview

The **goal** of individual and family* education is to improve individual health outcomes by promoting healthy behavior and appropriately involving individuals in their care† or services and in care decisions. Effective education will support recovery and speed optimal functioning. As appropriate to the care and services provided by the organization, care-related education involves

- facilitating the individual's or family's understanding of the individual's health status, health care options, and consequences of care or service choices;
- encouraging individual or family participation in the decision-making process about health care options;
- increasing the likelihood that the individual and family will follow the plan for care or services;
- maximizing the individual's independent living skills;
- increasing the individual's or family's ability to cope with the individual's health status, prognosis, or outcome;
- enhancing individual or family participation in continuing care or services;
- promoting healthy lifestyles;
- maintaining the individual's health status; and
- helping individuals and their families cope with death.

As appropriate to the care and services provided by the organization, academic education involves

- helping individuals and their families maintain ongoing academic education; and
- promoting academic knowledge and skill acquisition.

Education includes explaining psychiatric, physical, and functional diagnoses and prognoses to individuals and, when appropriate, families. Information about assessment and treatment options is communicated in a manner that facilitates understanding and elicits the individual's active participation in treatment planning.

Although standards in this chapter recommend a systematic approach to education throughout the organization, they do not prescribe any specific structure. Rather, they focus attention on the organization's current processes and whether they are consistent with the individual's plan of care, level of care or services, setting in which teaching occurs, and continuity of care or services.

---

* **family** The person(s) who plays a significant role in the member's life, which may include an individual(s) not legally related to the member. This person(s) is often referred to as a surrogate decision maker, if authorized to make care decisions for a member who loses decision-making capacity.

† "Care" includes individual care, treatment, services, rehabilitation, habilitation, or another program instituted for the individual served by the organization.

Standards

A list of all standards for this function appears below, presented without footnotes or other explanatory text. If you have any questions about a term used here, please refer to the standard as it appears in the next section of this chapter—Standards and Intent Statements.

PF.1 The organization plans, supports, and coordinates education activities and resources.

PF.2 Individuals and, when appropriate, their families receive education and training specific to the individuals' assessed needs, abilities, and readiness to learn, as appropriate to the care provided by the organization.

PF.2.1 Individuals and, when appropriate, their families are assessed on an ongoing basis to determine their learning needs, abilities, and readiness.

PF.2.1.1 When indicated, assessment of learning needs addresses cultural and religious beliefs, emotional barriers, desire and motivation to learn, physical or cognitive limitations, and barriers to communication.

PF.2.1.2 The knowledge, skills, and behaviors of individuals are assessed on an ongoing basis and, when appropriate, re-education is provided.

PF.2.2 Individualized instruction in the knowledge, skills, or behaviors required to meet ongoing health care needs is provided to individuals and families in ways that are understandable to them. Whenever appropriate, instruction is provided regarding

PF.2.2.1 safe and effective use of medication, in accordance with legal requirements and individual needs;

PF.2.2.2 the safe and effective use of medical equipment or supplies;

PF.2.2.3 potential drug-food interactions and nutrition intervention or modified diets;

PF.2.2.4 habilitation or rehabilitation techniques to facilitate adaptation to or functional independence in the environment;

PF.2.2.5 basic safety;

PF.2.2.6 access to available community resources; and

PF.2.2.7 resources available to meet the individual's identified needs.

PF.3 The organization identifies and provides the academic educational resources required to achieve its educational objectives.

PF.3.1 Academic education is provided to children and adolescents either directly by the organization or through other arrangements.

PF.4 Individual and family education is an interdisciplinary and coordinated process, as appropriate to the plan of care.

Standards and Intent Statements

Individual and Family Education and Responsibilities

Standard

PF.1 The organization plans, supports, and coordinates education activities and resources.

Intent of PF.1

Within its mission and scope of care and services, the organization plans and provides for individual and family education to promote and maintain health and improve care outcomes.

The organization considers

- the variety of settings in which individuals are taught;
- the types of individuals requiring education;
- the education materials available;
- the various staff members providing care or services; and
- the competence of staff who will teach individuals.

Standard

PF.2 Individuals and, when appropriate, their families receive education and training specific to the individuals' assessed needs, abilities, and readiness to learn, as appropriate to the care provided by the organization.

Intent of PF.2

Individual and family education is an integral part of providing care and services. The purpose of education is to teach skills, knowledge, and behaviors that promote recovery, maintain or improve function, or manage symptom progression. Positive outcomes often depend on

- the instructions given to an individual or family before they receive care or services; and
- information provided about health maintenance and improvement, tailored to the individual's health status.

The organization's overall framework for education is designed to help individuals or families gain the skills and knowledge necessary to meet ongoing needs. The process for identifying the individuals' learning and educational needs takes into account

- the scope of care and services provided by the organization;
- use of appropriate organization and community resources;
- the individual's or family's ability to understand and use the information taught; and
- the individual's or family's abilities and readiness for education.

Standards

PF.2.1 Individuals and, when appropriate, their families are assessed on an ongoing basis to determine their learning needs, abilities, and readiness.

PF.2.1.1 When indicated, assessment of learning needs addresses cultural and religious beliefs, emotional barriers, desire and motivation to learn, physical or cognitive limitations, and barriers to communication.

PF.2.1.2 The knowledge, skills, and behaviors of individuals are assessed on an ongoing basis and, when appropriate, re-education is provided.

Intent of PF.2.1 Through PF.2.1.2

Many variables have an impact on the effectiveness of education and the individual's or family's choices about following instructions. Being aware of these variables allows for openness and flexibility in teaching each individual and helps the organization determine appropriate educational methods and timing of educational activities. Therefore, all relevant data are collected and analyzed to determine individual and family learning needs, abilities, and readiness to learn. These assessments are conducted at intervals appropriate to the individual's care or service needs.

Based on the results of assessment, individual and family learning needs are prioritized. Staff members identify and teach skills and behaviors needed to optimize the individual's health outcomes.

The effectiveness of education is periodically assessed during the course of care. These assessments evaluate the individual's behaviors, performance of skills taught, and understanding of the information provided. When necessary, individuals are re-educated.

Standards

PF.2.2 *Individualized instruction in the knowledge, skills, or behaviors required to meet ongoing health care needs is provided to individuals and families in ways that are understandable to them. Whenever appropriate, instruction is provided regarding*

PF.2.2.1 safe and effective use of medication, in accordance with legal requirements and individual needs;

PF.2.2.2 the safe and effective use of medical equipment or supplies;

PF.2.2.3 potential drug-food interactions and nutrition intervention or modified diets;

PF.2.2.4 habilitation or rehabilitation techniques to facilitate adaptation to or functional independence in the environment;

PF.2.2.5 basic safety;

PF.2.2.6 access to available community resources; and

PF.2.2.7 resources available to meet the individual's identified needs.

Intent of PF.2.2 Through PF.2.2.7

Once the individual's learning needs are identified and prioritized, the educational process begins. Educational interventions are individualized to meet specific learning needs consistent with organization policies and procedures. Methods of education may include

- formal teaching plans;
- informal teaching opportunities; and
- demonstrations of skill or subject mastery by the individual or family.

Education in the safe and effective use of medication includes instruction in at least the name and description of the medication; the dosage, route of administration, and duration of drug therapy; special directions and precautions for the individual's preparation, self-administration, and use of the medication in the organization or at home, including safeguards against microbial contamination and appropriate compounding and administration techniques; intended use and expected actions of the drug therapy; common severe side effects,* adverse effects,† drug interactions and therapeutic contraindications, and how to avoid or respond to them; techniques for self-monitoring drug therapy; proper storage and expiration dating; prescription refill information; action in response to a missed dose; proper disposal of unused or expired medications, especially Schedule II drugs; and any other information relevant to the individual's particular needs or drug therapy.

When applicable, individuals or family members are informed of any infection prevention or control precautions to be taken, such as universal or barrier precautions. As appropriate, education services encompass health maintenance, including acquired immunodeficiency syndrome and sex education.

At the time of discharge, individuals in need of continuing care or services get written and verbal instruction about resources available to meet their continuing needs.

Academic Education

Standards

PF.3 The organization identifies and provides the academic educational resources required to achieve its educational objectives.

PF.3.1 Academic education is provided to children and adolescents either directly by the organization or through other arrangements.

Intent of PF.3 and PF.3.1

In keeping with its mission and scope of services, an organization must address the specific educational needs of individuals served either by directly providing services or through community resources, such as tutors or attendance at classes in public schools. When school-age children or adolescents are in the organization for long periods of time, state or local laws may specify the requirements for meeting the child's schooling needs. Although the organization may not provide school teachers directly, it is responsible for arranging schooling, according to state education law. An organization must provide or arrange for educational services, as needed by their specific populations. Adult education may be provided during an individual's stay or may be arranged through discharge and continuing-care planning.

* **side effect** A result of drug or other therapy in addition to or in extension of the desired therapeutic effect.

† **adverse effect** In pharmacology and therapeutics, the development of undesired side effects or toxicity due to the administration of drugs.

Educational resources are selected and provided to individuals based on their identified needs. The organization makes available educational services that

- provide special education experiences for individuals whose learning is hindered by their emotional condition or problems;
- help maintain the educational and intellectual development of all individuals served; and
- offer opportunities to catch up when individuals have fallen behind in their education because of their disorder.

Individuals are encouraged to take part in extracurricular school activities or community education programs when appropriate.

Individual and Family Education and Responsibilities

Standard

PF.4 Individual and family education is an interdisciplinary and coordinated process, as appropriate to the plan of care.

Intent of PF.4

To promote continuity and ensure that consistent information is provided to the individual and family, the education process is coordinated among the staff members providing care or services to the individual.

Educational resources are selected based on the individual's or, when appropriate, family's educational needs. For each individual or family, education incorporates appropriate

- members of the care team;
- types of materials;
- methods of teaching;
- community educational resources, if needed, particularly for the academic education of children and adolescents; and
- special devices, interpreters, or other aids to meet specialized needs.

Continuum

Overview

The **goal** of the continuum function is to provide care appropriate to individual needs in a continuous and coordinated manner within and among settings. Health care organizations must view the care they provide as part of a continuum that over time gives individuals access to an integrated system of settings, services, and care levels. When making care and services available, organization leaders consider the needs of the populations served, available resources, strategies, and settings for delivery of service. Channels of communication among service providers facilitate stability, continuity, and comprehensiveness of services to each individual.

Within the continuum of care,* each organization defines, shapes, and sequences the following processes and activities to maximize coordination of care†:

Before Admission

- Information is collected from various sources, including other organizations or programs, and used to identify individuals' needs.
- Links are made with other organizations or programs.

During Admission

- Services are made available consistent with the organization's mission, population, and treatment settings or services to meet identified needs.
- Arrangements are made with other organizations and settings to facilitate entry.
- Referrals‡ and transfers§ are made and clinical consultants or contractual arrangements are used to meet individuals' needs.

Within the Organization

- Care and services flow continuously from assessment through treatment and reassessment.
- Care and services are coordinated among clinicians and programs.

Before Exit

- Individuals' status and need for continuing care** are assessed.

---

* **continuum of care** Matching the individual's ongoing needs with the appropriate level and type of physical, psychological, or social services.

† **coordination of care** Integration of the components of care.

‡ **referral** The sending of an individual (1) from one clinician to another clinician or specialist, (2) from one setting or service to another, or (3) by one physician (the referring physician) to another physician (or some other resource) either for consultation or care.

§ **transfer** The formal shifting of responsibility for the care of an individual (1) from one care unit to another, (2) from one clinical service to another, or (3) from the care of one licensed independent practitioner to another.

** **continuing care** Care provided over an extended time, in various settings, spanning the continuum of health and functioning.

At Exit

- Individuals are referred directly to practitioners, programs, and organizations to meet their continuing needs.
- Need for continuing care is reassessed.
- Information is provided to help others meet individuals' continuing needs.

Other functional areas that support continuum of care include leadership's planning and management of services, assessment, education, and management of information.

The continuum function is the heart of case management. The standards in this chapter especially apply to case-management services.

Standards

A list of all standards for this function appears below, presented without footnotes or other explanatory text. If you have any questions about a term used here, please refer to the standard as it appears in the next section of this chapter—Standards and Intent Statements.

CC.1 Within its capability, the organization has a process to provide access to the appropriate level of care, health professionals, programs, and services to meet individuals' assessed needs.

CC.2 Individuals are accepted for entry to appropriate services or programs based on intake, assessment, and transfer procedures.

CC.2.1 Criteria define the information necessary to determine an individual's eligibility for entry to a program or service.

CC.3 As appropriate to the settings of care, the services provided, and the individual's condition, individuals and, when appropriate, families receive enough information to make knowledgeable decisions about care and services. Information provided includes

CC.3.1 the nature and goals of care and services;

CC.3.2 the hours during which care and services are available;

CC.3.3 the costs of care and services to be borne by the individual, if any;

CC.3.4 the individual's rights, responsibilities, and involvement in care; and

CC.3.5 arranging for dependent care services, if necessary, while the individual is in treatment.

CC.4 The organization provides for continuity of care and services over time among the assessment and diagnosis, planning, and treatment phases of the individual's services.

CC.5 The organization provides for coordination of care and services among health professionals and settings.

CC.6 Referral, transfer, or discharge of individuals to other levels of care, health professionals, or settings are based on individuals' assessed needs and the organization's capability to provide needed care.

CC.6.1 The discharge process provides for continuing care to meet the individual's assessed needs at the time of discharge.

CC.6.1.1 The individual is informed in a timely manner of the need for planning for discharge or transfer to another organization or level of care.

CC.7 Appropriate care and clinical information is exchanged when individuals are admitted, referred, transferred, or discharged to receive further care or services.

CC.8 If an external entity conducts a utilization review to determine the appropriateness of admissions, continuation of current care, or specific care and services, and that review results in denial of care, services, or payment, then decisions regarding provision of ongoing care and services or discharge continue to be based on the identified needs of the individual being served.

Standards and Intent Statements

Continuum

Standard

CC.1 Within its capability, the organization has a process to provide access to the appropriate level of care, health professionals, programs, and services to meet individuals' assessed needs.

Intent of CC.1

Individuals are screened at the point of first contact with the organization. After screening, individuals are matched with the services or programs within the organization that are most appropriate to their needs. The organization's decision to provide a specific service or program is based on its mission and capability to provide the requisite staffing, facilities, and services.

Various processes can be designed to ensure individuals gain access to appropriate care on a timely basis. The organization defines what information should be gathered during the screening to determine admission or referral. (See the "Assessment" chapter of this manual [page 61].)

Standard

CC.2 Individuals are accepted for entry* to appropriate services or programs based on intake, assessment, and transfer procedures.†

Intent of CC.2

To facilitate the delivery of appropriate, effective care and service, the organization designs a procedure that addresses the entry process. The procedure includes intake, assessment, and transfer procedures to ensure that acceptance of the individual is appropriate.

Standard

CC.2.1 Criteria define the information necessary to determine an individual's eligibility for entry to a program or service.

Intent of CC.2.1

The organization defines the minimum essential information needed to determine an individual's eligibility for entry to a setting or program. The criteria are based on the specific program or service that can meet or respond to the needs or presenting conditions of the individual. To add clarity, entry criteria also include exclusionary statements that indicate the information needed to initiate referral to another, more appropriate program or organization.

---

* **entry** The process by which an individual is screened and/or assessed by the organization's setting, service, or program in order to determine the organization's capabilities to provide the care or rehabilitation services appropriate to the individual's needs.

† **intake, assessment, and transfer procedures** The processes an organization establishes by which appropriate and necessary information is obtained for each individual seeking entry into a health care setting or service. The information is used to match individual needs with the level of care required and to the appropriate setting.

Standards

CC.3 *As appropriate to the settings of care, the services provided, and the individual's condition, individuals and, when appropriate, families* receive enough information to make knowledgeable decisions about care and services. Information provided includes*

CC.3.1 the nature and goals of care and services;

CC.3.2 the hours during which care and services are available;

CC.3.3 the costs of care and services to be borne by the individual, if any;

CC.3.4 the individual's rights, responsibilities, and involvement in care; and

CC.3.5 arranging for dependent care services, if necessary, while the individual is in treatment.

Intent of CC.3 Through CC.3.5

Requirements for entry to settings or services are clearly communicated to individuals and, when appropriate, to their families.† They are given enough information about the care or services to make a knowledgeable decision about whether to seek them. Insurance coverage and managed care arrangements are explained as part of this process.

Due to the practices of health insurance and managed health care, insurance reviewers, managed care utilization reviewers, and case-management professionals may contribute to clinical decisions about an individual's treatment (including type of care and the clinical necessity for care). These individuals and their employers may work with the clinician in developing the least restrictive and most cost-sensitive treatment plan.

Individuals and, as appropriate, their families should be aware that treatment may be shortened or modified. The individuals served and clinicians always have the right to appeal any funding decisions regarding treatment (see CC.8).

Standards

CC.4 The organization provides for continuity of care and services over time among the assessment and diagnosis, planning, and treatment phases of the individual's services.

CC.5 The organization provides for coordination of care and services among health professionals and settings.

Intent of CC.4 and CC.5

Processes for assessing, planning for, and meeting individuals' health care needs promote smooth transitions from one level of care to the next. Throughout care, individuals are matched with appro-

---

* **family** The person(s) who plays a significant role in the member's life, which may include an individual(s) not legally related to the member. This person(s) is often referred to as a surrogate decision maker, if authorized to make care decisions for a member who loses decision-making capacity.

† When the term "individuals or their families" or a variation of it is used in this manual, it takes into consideration the rights of the individual served to exercise personal privacy by withholding consent for participation in care and service decisions of family members or significant others.

priate resources within the continuum (for example, crisis stabilization units, residential care, supervised housing). Services are coordinated to ensure appropriate continuity of care from the time of entry through assessment, planning, treatment, and discharge. Delivery of services to meet each individual's set of biopsychosocial needs is integrated and responsive to changing needs.

Standard

CC.6 Referral, transfer, or discharge of individuals to other levels of care, health professionals, or settings are based on individuals' assessed needs and the organization's capability to provide needed care.

Intent of CC.6

Transfer, referral, or discharge processes address

- shifting responsibility for an individual's care from one clinician, organization, organizational unit or clinical service to another (which could include transferring complete responsibility for the individual and his or her care to others or referring the individual to others, such as one or more agencies or professionals, to provide one or more specific services);
- the reason for transfer, referral, or discharge;
- the conditions under which transfer can occur (for example, the individual is not transferred until the receiving organization has consented to accept the individual and the individual is considered sufficiently stabilized);
- responsibility for the individual during transfer; and
- procedures for internal and external referral.

Referrals can be made through formal affiliations or informal arrangements by placement contacts.

Standard

CC.6.1 The discharge process provides for continuing care to meet the individual's assessed needs at the time of discharge.

Intent of CC.6.1

For some individuals, effective discharge planning addresses how needs will be met as they move to the next level of care. For other individuals, discharge planning will consist of a clear understanding of how to access services in the future should the need arise. Planning identifies individuals' post-discharge needs (for example, physical, emotional, housekeeping, transportation, social), and helps arrange for services to meet those needs. Some options to meet discharge needs include special education, adult foster care, case management, home health services, hospice care, long term care facilities, ambulatory care, support groups, and rehabilitation facilities.

The discharge-planning process involves, as appropriate, the licensed independent practitioner primarily responsible for care management, other appropriate staff, the individual, and the individual's family or significant other. To facilitate continuity of care after discharge, the individual and, when appropriate, the family and/or significant other are assisted in adapting to the care plan.

Standard

CC.6.1.1 The individual is informed in a timely manner of the need for planning for discharge or transfer to another organization or level of care.

Intent of CC.6.1.1

The organization is responsible for keeping the individual and the individual's family informed of the care process, especially when the organization anticipates some level of care continuing after discharge. These discussions begin as early as possible in the care process, continue throughout it, and include the anticipated time of discharge. Individual and family education and continuity of care are related functions. This relationship is clear in the discharge-planning process, which includes giving the individual and family information about

- the conditions that may result in transfer to another organization or level of care;
- alternatives to transfer, if any;
- the clinical basis for discharge; and
- the anticipated need for continued care following discharge.

Standard

CC.7 Appropriate care and clinical information is exchanged when individuals are admitted, referred, transferred, or discharged to receive further care or services.

Intent of CC.7

The individual may receive health care in many settings or services and may be referred from one organization or provider to another. To facilitate continuity of care, appropriate information is communicated to any health care organization or provider to which the individual is admitted, referred, transferred, or discharged. Tracking an individual's care with consistent information makes service coordination easier within the organization, among various other organizations, and among services within the community.

For the accepting organization to meet the individual's needs, the following information is exchanged:

- The reason for transfer, referral, or discharge;
- Relevant biopsychosocial status at the time of transfer, referral, or discharge;
- A summary of the care or service provided and progress toward achieving goals; and
- Instruction and names of referrals given to the individual.

Standard

CC.8 If an external entity conducts a utilization review to determine the appropriateness of admissions, continuation of current care, or specific care and services, and that review results in denial of care, services, or payment, then decisions regarding provision of ongoing care and services or discharge continue to be based on the identified needs of the individual being served.

Intent of CC.8

Once individuals request or present themselves for treatment or service, the organization is professionally and ethically responsible for providing care within its capability, mission, and applicable law and regulation. At times, indications for such care may contradict the recommendations of an external entity conducting utilization review (for example, peer review organizations, insurance companies, or managed-care reviewers). If such a conflict arises, treatment and discharge decisions must be made in response to the care required by the individual, regardless of the external agency's recommendation. The organization involves the individual and, as appropriate, the individual's family in deliberations about the denial of care or conflict about care decisions.

Improving Organization Performance

Overview

The **goal** of the improving organization performance function is that the organization designs processes well and systematically monitors, analyzes, and improves its performance to improve individual outcomes. Value in behavioral health care is the appropriate balance between good outcomes, excellent care and services, and costs. In order to add value to the care and services provided, organizations need to understand the relation between perception of care, outcomes, and costs and how these three issues are affected by processes carried out by the organization. An organization's performance of important functions significantly affects the quality and value of its services.

The organization's approach to improving its performance includes the following essential processes:

- Designing processes,
- Monitoring performance through data collection,
- Analyzing current performance, and
- Improving and sustaining improved performance.

This approach is anchored in the real work of health care professionals and in the real improvements that can be achieved to benefit individuals and others.

Because most organizations identify more improvement opportunities than they can act on, priorities have to be set. Criteria are helpful in setting priorities and can include

- the expected impact on performance;
- selecting high-risk, high-volume, or problem-prone processes to monitor;
- the relationship of the potential improvement to the dimensions of performance and functions in this manual; and
- the organization's resources.

All relevant disciplines participate in testing or implementing improvement strategies. After such implementation, the success of the new strategy is again measured.

Continuously monitoring, analyzing, and improving performance of clinical and other processes are the heart of this function and what the standards in this chapter address. Leaders* and staff carry out these activities. Examples of improvement efforts include designing a new service, flowcharting a clinical process, collecting data about performance measures or individual outcomes, comparing the organization's performance to that of other organizations, selecting areas for priority attention, and even experimenting with new ways of carrying out a function.

Leadership also empowers and assigns an individual to lead the improvement by providing time and resources necessary to make the improvement throughout the organization.

---

* **Leader** An individual who sets expectations, develops plans, and implements procedures to assess and improve the quality of the organization's governance, management, clinical, and support functions. Leaders include at least members of the governing body; the chief executive officer and other senior managers; clinical leaders (clinical leaders include health care professionals with overall responsibility to plan, organize, and operate a clinical service or program and may include but are not limited to the clinical director, discipline chief, and unit or service director); and staff members in a leadership position within the organization.

Dimensions of Performance

Performance is *what* is done and *how well* it is done to provide health care. The level of performance in health care is

- the degree to which *what* is done is *efficacious* and *appropriate* for the individual; and
- the degree to which it is *available* in a *timely* manner to individuals who need it, *effective, continuous* with other care and care providers, *safe, efficient,* and *caring* and *respectful* of the individual.

Characteristics of *what* is done and *how well* it is done are called *dimensions of performance.* These characteristics include:

- The degree to which an organization does the right things and does them well is influenced strongly by its design and operation of a number of important functions—many of which are described in this manual.
- The effect of an organization's performance of these functions is reflected in individual outcomes and in the cost of its services.
- Individuals and others judge the quality of the health care based on individual health outcomes (and sometimes on their perceptions of what was done and how it was done).
- Individuals and others may also judge the value of the health care by comparing their judgments about quality with the cost of the health care.

The dimensions of performance are defined in Table 1 (below).

Table 1. Dimensions of Performance

I. Doing the Right Thing

The **efficacy** of the procedure or treatment in relation to the individual's condition

> The degree to which the individual's care and services have been shown to accomplish the desired or projected outcome(s)

The **appropriateness** of a specific test, procedure, or service to meet the individual's needs

> The degree to which the care and services provided are relevant to the individual's clinical needs, given the current state of knowledge

II. Doing the Right Thing Well

The **availability** of a needed test, procedure, treatment, or service to the individual who needs it

> The degree to which appropriate care and services are available to meet the individual's needs

The **timeliness** with which a needed test, procedure, treatment, or service is provided to the individual

> The degree to which the care and services are provided to the individual at the most beneficial or necessary time

The **effectiveness** with which tests, procedures, treatments, and services are provided

> The degree to which the care and services are provided in the correct manner, given the current state of knowledge, to achieve the desired or projected outcome for the individual

Table 1. Dimensions of Performance (continued)

The **continuity** of the services provided to the individual with respect to other services, practitioners, and providers and over time

> The degree to which the individual's care is coordinated among disciplines, among organizations, and over time

The **safety** of the individual and others to whom the services are provided

> The degree to which the risk of an intervention and risk in the care environment are reduced for the individual and others, including the health care provider

The **efficiency** with which care and services are provided

> The relationship between the outcomes (results of care) and the resources used to deliver individual care and services

The **respect and caring** with which care and services are provided

> The degree to which those providing care and services do so with sensitivity and respect for the individual's needs, expectations, and individual differences
>
> The degree to which the individual or a designee is involved in his or her own care and service decisions

Standards

A list of standards for this function appears below, presented without footnotes or other explanatory text. If you have any questions about a term used here, please refer to the standard as it appears in the next section of this chapter—Standards and Intent Statements.

PI.1 The leaders establish a planned, systematic, organizationwide approach to process design and performance measurement, analysis, and improvement.

PI.1.1 The activities are planned in a collaborative and interdisciplinary manner.

PI.2 New or modified processes are designed well.

PI.2.1 Performance expectations are established for new and modified processes.

PI.2.2 The performance of new and modified processes is measured.

PI.3 Data are collected to monitor the stability of existing processes, identify opportunities for improvement, identify changes that will lead to improvement, and sustain improvements.

PI.3.1 The organization collects data to monitor its performance.

PI.3.1.1 The organization collects data to monitor the performance of processes that involve risks or may result in sentinel events.

PI.3.1.2 The organization collects data to monitor performance of areas targeted for further study.

PI.3.1.3 The organization collects data to monitor improvements in performance.

PI.4 Data are systematically aggregated and analyzed on an ongoing basis.

PI.4.1 Appropriate statistical techniques are used to analyze and display data.

PI.4.2 The organization compares its performance over time and with other sources of information.

PI.4.3 Undesirable patterns or trends in performance and sentinel events are intensively analyzed.

PI.4.4 The organization identifies changes that will lead to improved performance and reduce the risk of sentinel events.

PI.5 Improved performance is achieved and sustained.

Standards and Intent Statements

Design

Leadership Role in Improving Organization Performance

If an organization is to initiate and maintain improvement, leadership and planning are essential. This is especially critical for uniting existing and new improvement activities into a systematic, organizationwide approach. These standards point to the importance of leadership's role in planning an approach to improvement. In conjunction with standards in the "Leadership" chapter, the leaders also ensure that necessary processes and structures are in place to carry out performance improvement activities and that all services and disciplines collaborate to carry out that approach.

Standards

PI.1 *The leaders establish a planned, systematic, organizationwide approach to process design and performance measurement, analysis, and improvement.*

PI.1.1 *The activities are planned in a collaborative and interdisciplinary manner.*

Intent of PI.1 and PI.1.1

Performance improvement activities are most effective when they are planned, systematic, and organizationwide and all appropriate individuals and professions work collaboratively to plan and implement them. At times, performance improvement efforts do occur within specific departments, units, or disciplines. This happens when the organization is small in size or when the services of only one distinct discipline are provided. However, when the disciplines representing the scope of care and services across the organization are included in performance improvement activities, complex problems and processes can be improved. The ongoing mutual support that develops among interdisciplinary groups provides the momentum necessary to complete long-term improvement projects. Collaboration on performance improvement activities enables an organization to create a culture focused on performance improvement and to plan and provide systematic and organizationwide improvement.

Standard

PI.2 New or modified processes are designed well.

Intent of PI.2

When processes, functions, or services are designed well, they draw on a variety of information sources. Good process design

a. is consistent with the organization's mission, vision, values, goals and objectives, and plans;
b. meets the needs of individuals served, staff, and others;
c. is clinically sound and current (for instance, use of practice guidelines, information from relevant literature, and clinical standards);
d. is consistent with sound business practices;

e. incorporates available information from other organizations about occurrence of sentinel events* in order to reduce the risk of similar sentinel events; and

f. incorporates the results of performance improvement activities.

The organization incorporates information related to these elements, when available and relevant, in the design or redesign of processes, functions, or services.

Standards

PI.2.1 Performance expectations are established for new and modified processes.

PI.2.2 The performance of new and modified processes is measured.

Intent of PI.2.1 and PI.2.2

Performance expectations† are identified during the design or redesign phase of a function, process, or service. A performance measure‡ is used to determine if the process, function, or service is actually performing according to the identified performance expectations and the way it was designed. Performance measures can be developed by the organization or be adopted or adapted from measure sets used in existing databases, which will enable data collection and comparison between or among locations or organizations.

The organization uses criteria to define their own performance measures or to select performance measures from an external system. The criteria help ensure that the data collected are appropriate for monitoring performance. The criteria include the following:

- The measure can identify the events it was intended to identify;
- The measure has a documented numerator and a denominator statement or description of the population to which the measure is applicable;
- The measure has defined data elements and allowable values;
- The measure can detect changes in performance over time;
- The measure allows for comparison over time within the organization or between the organization and other entities (this may require risk adjustment);
- The data intended for collection are available; and
- Results can be reported in a way that is useful to the organization and other interested stakeholders.

The performance measures are the benchmarks or statistical measures to be used for comparison.

---

* **sentinel event** A sentinel event is an unexpected occurrence involving death or serious physical or psychological injury, or risk thereof. Serious injury specifically includes loss of life or function. The phrase "or the risk thereof" includes any process variation for which a recurrence would carry a significant chance of a serious adverse outcome.

† Performance expectations are attributes or dimensions (such as timeliness, effectiveness, and efficiency) which describe expected performance of a function, process, or service. They define how something is expected to work.

‡ **performance measure** A quantitative tool that provides an indication of an organization's performance in relation to a specified process or outcome.

Data Collection

Monitoring Performance Through Data Collection

Monitoring performance through data collection is the foundation of all performance improvement activities. Collecting data about current performance provides for such information and allows the organization to

- make informed judgments about the stability* of existing processes (for example, undesirable process variation);
- identify opportunities for incrementally improving processes;
- identify the need to redesign processes; and
- decide if improvements or redesign of processes meet objectives.

Because most organizations have limited resources, they cannot collect data to monitor everything they want to monitor. Leaders must therefore decide which processes to monitor and the data to be collected. They determine the importance of the organization's processes in relation to its mission, available resources, and functions, as well as concerns of the individuals served, their families, staff, payers, and other customers.

Data collection focuses on

- processes, particularly those that are high risk, high volume, or problem prone;
- outcomes;
- targeted areas of study;
- comprehensive performance measures (indicators);
- other gauges of performance such as
  - clients' and others' needs, expectations, and feedback,
  - results of ongoing infection control activities,
  - safety of the environment, and
  - quality control and risk-management findings; and
- the dimensions of performance (such as efficiency and timeliness) that are important to a process or an outcome.

The organization's leaders decide the scope and focus of performance monitoring and data collection activities. In determining the scope, the leaders identify and consider the important care and services and organization functions performed. The important functions common to all health care organizations are identified by the chapter titles in this manual and represent logical starting points. The leaders determine the focus of data collection monitoring when they set priorities for monitoring. In setting priorities, they consider and are guided by various concerns, such as identified high-risk or problem-prone processes or results from regulatory or accreditation reports. An organizationwide approach to monitoring performance will, over time, include measures that relate to each of the important functions described in this manual.

Once they determine the scope and focus of monitoring and data collection, the leaders decide

- how to organize those activities into a systematic approach;
- the frequency and intensity of data collection;
- the relevant dimensions of performance to be monitored; and
- the incorporation of data collection activities into daily work processes.

---

* A stable process can have very large common-cause variation or can fail to produce the desired results. So it is possible to have a process that is stable, yet incapable of performing satisfactorily.

The standards in this chapter allow each organization to develop its own approach and are therefore equally applicable to approaches that organize monitoring and data collection around clinical paths, product lines, or important functions. Finally, some processes are measured on a periodic, ongoing basis while other processes are measured more intensively.

Standard

PI.3 *Data are collected to monitor the stability of existing processes, identify opportunities for improvement, identify changes that will lead to improvement, and sustain improvement.*

Intent for PI.3

Collected data help the organization evaluate outcomes or determine the performance of a function or process. When data collection is systematic, it can be used to

- establish a performance baseline;
- describe process performance or stability;
- describe the dimensions of performance relevant to functions, processes, and outcomes;
- identify areas for more focused data collection; and
- sustain improvement.

The leaders use the judgments made about stability or performance to identify and prioritize issues for more focused data collection and analysis (see LD.4.2.2 and LD.4.3 for the leaders using criteria to prioritize data collection for improvement).

Standard

PI.3.1 The organization collects data to monitor its performance.

Intent for PI.3.1

Performance monitoring and improvement are data driven. The stability of important processes can provide the organization with information about its performance. Every organization must choose which processes and outcomes (and thus types of data) are important to monitor based on its mission and the scope of care and services provided. The leaders prioritize data collection based on the organization's mission, care and services provided, and populations served (see LD.4.2.2 for priority setting). Data that the organization considers for collection to monitor performance include the following:

- Performance measures related to accreditation and other requirements;
- Risk management;
- Utilization management;
- Quality control;
- Staff opinions and needs;
- Behavior management* procedures, if used;
- Outcomes of processes or services;
- Performance measures from acceptable databases;
- Customer demographics and diagnoses;
- Financial data;
- Infection control surveillance and reporting;

* The use of basic learning techniques, such as biofeedback, reinforcement, or aversion therapy, to manage and improve an individual's behavior.

- Research data; and
- Performance data identified in various chapters of this manual.

For all organizations the following data are required to be collected:

- the needs, expectations, and satisfaction of individuals* and organizations served; individuals served and family members can provide information to give an organization insight about process design and functioning. The organization asks them about
  - their specific needs and expectations;
  - their perceptions of how well the organization meets these needs and expectations; and
  - how the organization can improve.

The organization can use a number of ways to get input from these groups including perception-of-care surveys, regularly scheduled meetings held with these groups, and focus groups.

The detail and frequency of data collection are determined as appropriate for monitoring ongoing performance. Data are collected at the frequency and with the detail identified by the organization. When possible, data collection is incorporated into day-to-day activities rather than as a separate activity.

Standard

PI.3.1.1 The organization collects data to monitor the performance of processes that involve risks or may result in sentinel events.

Intent of PI.3.1.1

Organizations select processes which are known to be high-risk, high-volume, problem-prone areas related to the care and services provided. This information is correlated with the listing of frequently-occurring sentinel events published by the Joint Commission, the organization's risk-management data, or information about problematic processes generated by field-specific or professional organizations.

Organizations select performance measures for processes known to jeopardize the safety of the individuals served or are associated with sentinel events in similar health care organizations. At a minimum, the organization identifies performance measures related to the following processes as appropriate to the care and services provided:

- Medication use;
- Operative and other procedures† that place individuals at risk;
- Use of blood and blood components;
- Restraint use;
- Seclusion; and
- Care or services provided to high-risk populations.

The detail and frequency of data collection have been determined and are appropriate for monitoring high-risk, problem-prone processes. Data are collected at the frequency and with the detail identified by the organization.

The performance measure data are used to evaluate outcomes or performance of problem-prone processes.

---

* In order to better measure the performance of organizations regarding how well they meet the needs, expectations and concerns of individuals, the Joint Commission is moving from the term satisfaction toward the more inclusive term perception of care and service. By using this term, the organization will be prompted to assess not only the individuals' and/or families' satisfaction with care or treatment, but also whether their needs and expectations are met by the organization.

† Includes operative, other invasive, and noninvasive procedures that place the individual at risk. In this context, the focus is on procedures and is not meant to include medications that place the individual at risk.

Standard

PI.3.1.2 The organization collects data to monitor performance of areas targeted for further study.

Intent of PI.3.1.2

A specific area for further study is identified by considering the information provided by the data about process stability, risks, and sentinel events, and priorities set by the leaders. Narrowing the focus of study allows the organization to better describe processes related to the area of study, allows data collection to occur as processes are carried out and allows the organization to identify potential changes that can lead to more significant improvement. The targeted area for further study can be a specific population, a specific diagnosis, a specific service provided, or an organization management issue and is time limited. Performance measures are chosen which address the topic area.

The detail and frequency of data collection are determined as appropriate for monitoring targeted areas of study. Data are collected at the frequency and with the detail identified by the organization. The data collected about the performance measures help focus change or improvement activities for that specific area of study.

Standard

PI.3.1.3 The organization collects data to monitor improvements in performance.

Intent of PI.3.1.3

When planning for improvement, the organization identifies those areas needing improvement and identifies the desired changes (see PI.4.4). Performance measures are then identified in order to determine whether the change results in an improvement and value is increased. Data are collected on the performance measures. The data are analyzed to determine the effectiveness of the change. Performance measures are used on a continuing basis to ensure continued improvement once the change is fully implemented. Data are collected for a period of time that allows the organization to ensure that sustained improvement continues.

If a process is redesigned as part of an improvement activity, then data are collected for the performance measures that were developed as part of the redesign activity.

The detail and frequency of data collection have been determined and are appropriate for monitoring improvements in performance. For example, data collection may be ongoing or time limited. Data are collected at the frequency and with the detail identified by the organization.

Aggregation and Analysis

Aggregating and Analyzing Data to Support Performance Improvement

Aggregating and analyzing data means transforming that data into information. The organization can use this information to draw conclusions about its performance of a process or the nature of the outcome. Data analysis can answer questions such as the following:

- What is our current level of performance?
- How stable are our current processes?

- Are there areas that could be improved?
- Was a strategy to stabilize or improve performance effective?
- Did we meet design specifications for processes?

The goal is to develop an analysis process that incorporates four basic comparisons: with self, with other similar behavioral health care organizations, with standards, and with best practices. How often the organization aggregates and analyzes data depends on the process being measured and the organization's priorities. For example, an organization might analyze data about the medication reactions every month and data about staff-education needs every six months.

Conclusions about current performance based on data analysis may indicate a need for targeted study or more intense analysis of processes or outcomes. Such conclusions are based on comparison with

- preestablished criteria;
- sentinel events;
- control limits;*
- review of all occurrences; or
- other interpretation methods.

Data analysis is interdisciplinary when appropriate for the process or outcome under review. When the analysis focuses on an individual's clinical performance, the organization takes appropriate action.

Standard

PI.4 Data are systematically aggregated and analyzed on an ongoing basis.

Intent of PI.4

The frequency with which data are aggregated has been determined and is appropriate to the activity or area being studied. Aggregation of data at ongoing points in time enables the organization to judge a particular process's stability or a particular outcome's predictability in relation to performance expectations. Aggregated data are analyzed in order to make judgments about

- whether design specifications for processes were met;
- the level of performance and stability of important existing processes;
- opportunities for improvement;
- actions to improve the performance of processes; and
- whether changes in the processes resulted in improvement.

Standard

PI.4.1 Appropriate statistical techniques are used to analyze and display data.

Intent of PI.4.1

Understanding statistical techniques are helpful in both assessing variation and studying a process to determine where the improvement needs to occur. By understanding the type and cause of variation through use of statistical tools and methods, the organization can focus its attention and resources on making improvement changes to those processes which will result in better outcomes. Some of the types of statistical tools which could be considered are

---

* **control limits** In statistics, an expected limit of common-cause variation, sometimes referred to as either an upper or a lower limit. Variation beyond a control limit is evidence that special causes are affecting a process. Control limits are calculated from process data and are not to be confused with engineering specifications or tolerance limits. Control limits are typically plotted on a control chart.

- run charts which display summary and comparative data;
- control charts which display variation and trends over time;
- histograms;
- Pareto charts;
- cause-and-effect or fishbone diagrams; and
- other statistical tools as appropriate.

Standard

PI.4.2 The organization compares its performance over time and with other sources of information.

Intent of PI.4.2

Performance can be evaluated from three perspectives:

- Performance compared internally over time;
- Performance compared to performance of similar processes in other organizations; and
- Performance compared to external sources of information.

These comparisons are used to determine if there is excessive variability or unacceptable levels of performance of processes and outcomes.

External sources are as up-to-date as possible and include

- recent scientific, clinical, and management literature;
- well-formulated practice guidelines or parameters;
- performance measures;
- reference databases; and
- standards that are periodically reviewed and revised.

Reference databases are excellent sources of performance information. They permit comparison with like process and outcomes in other organizations and may lead to identifying best practices. Organizations that collect long-term data about the individuals served use the data, as appropriate, to improve themselves.

Standard

PI.4.3 Undesirable patterns or trends in performance and sentinel events are intensively analyzed.

Intent of PI.4.3

When the organization detects or suspects significant undesirable performance or variation, it initiates intense analysis to determine where best to focus changes for improvement. The organization initiates intense analysis when the comparisons show that

- important single events, levels of performance, patterns, or trends vary significantly and undesirably from those expected;
- performance varies significantly and undesirably from that of other organizations;
- performance varies significantly and undesirably from recognized standards; or
- when a sentinel event occurs.

When monitoring performance of specific clinical processes, certain events always elicit intense analysis. Based on the scope of care or services provided, intense analysis is performed for the following:

- Significant adverse drug reactions; and
- Significant medication errors.*

Intense analysis can also occur for those topics chosen by the leaders as performance-improvement priorities or when undesirable variation occurs which changes the priorities. Of course, an organization may also initiate further analysis at any time to improve its current performance. Intense analysis involves studying a process to learn in greater detail about how it is performed or how it operates.

A root cause analysis† is performed for a sentinel event occurrence.

Standard

PI.4.4 The organization identifies changes that will lead to improved performance and reduce the risk of sentinel events.

Intent of PI.4.4

The organization uses the information from the data analysis to identify changes that will improve performance or reduce the risk of sentinel events. Changes are identified based on the analysis of data from targeted study or from analysis of data from ongoing monitoring. A change is selected, and the organization plans to implement the change on a pilot test basis or across the organization. Performance measures are selected that help determine the effectiveness of the change and whether it resulted in an improvement (see PI.3.1.1, PI.3.1.2, and PI.3.1.3) once the change is implemented.

Performance Improvement

Performance Improvement

The purpose of the performance improvement function is to improve existing processes and outcomes and then sustain the improved performance. This can be accomplished by incrementally improving existing processes, redesigning an existing process, or designing an essentially new process (for example, re-engineering).

Leaders recognize and celebrate improvement successes. To sustain improvements, leaders support one-on-one discussions among professionals and other staff of successful changes. Change is managed and implemented incrementally.

Standard

PI.5 Improved performance is achieved and sustained.

---

* **significant medication errors and significant adverse drug reactions** Unintended, undesirable and unexpected effects of prescribed medications or of medication errors that require discontinuing a medication or modifying the dose, require initial or prolonged hospitalization, result in disability, require treatment with a prescription medication, result in cognitive deterioration or impairment, are life threatening, result in death, or result in congenital anomalies.

† **root cause analysis** A process for identifying the basic or causal factor(s) that underlie variation in performance, including the occurrence or possible occurrence of a sentinel event.

Intent of PI.5

Once performance improvement priorities are identified, the organization uses appropriate resources and involves those individuals, disciplines, and departments closest to the process, function, or service identified for improvement. Changes to improve performance are identified, planned, and tested. Effective changes are incorporated into standard operating procedure.

The organization sustains improvement through education of key staff about the redesigned process(es) or other changes being implemented. Their input is obtained as they begin to carry out the process to identify additional opportunities for improvements. Performance measures are used (see PI.2.2, PI.3.1.2, and PI.3.1.3) to determine if the improvement is sustained. Data are collected as part of performance monitoring. Feedback is provided to staff and leaders on a regular basis.

The organization reduces the risk of sentinel events by using available information about sentinel events known to occur with significant frequency in health care organizations that provide similar care and services. This is done so that the organization can design or redesign care and services to prevent the event from occurring in its organization.

Leadership

Overview

The **goal** of the leadership function is to improve individual care and services, as well as outcomes, through effective leadership. The organization's leaders* play a critical role in delivering care and services† that are responsive to individual and community needs. The organization's leaders lay the foundation for planning, directing, coordinating, providing, and improving care and services throughout the organization.

Key Characteristics of Leadership

Leadership begins with establishing and communicating the organization's mission, vision, and values and, when necessary, reviewing and revising them. Building on the organization's mission, the leaders articulate a clear vision for the future and define the values that underlie all day-to-day activities throughout the organization. Effective leadership

- defines a strategic plan consistent with the organization's mission, vision, and values;
- clearly communicates the mission, vision, values, and strategic plan throughout the organization;
- accurately assesses the needs of individuals served by the organization as well as the needs of other users of the organization's services;
- encourages staff participation in the organization's development;
- assumes an active role in teaching staff; and
- develops leaders at every level of the organization to help fulfill the organization's mission, vision, and values.

By providing the proper direction, coordination, culture, and resources, the leaders establish a framework for realizing the organization's strategic goals and vision. This framework guides implementation and improvement of services throughout the organization.

The Processes of Leadership

To achieve the goal of the leadership function, the following four processes must be performed well:

1. **Planning for services.** Leadership develops a mission statement and ensures it is reflected in all long-range, strategic and operational plans, resource allocation, and organizational policies.
2. **Directing services.** Leadership organizes, directs, and staffs care‡ and services commensurate with the scope of services offered.
3. **Implementing and coordinating services.** Leadership integrates care and services throughout the organization.

---

* **leader** An individual who sets expectations, develops plans, and implements procedures to assess and improve the quality of the organization's governance, management, clinical, and support functions. Leaders include at least members of the governing body; the chief executive officer and other senior managers; clinical leaders (clinical leaders include health care professionals with overall responsibility to plan, organize, and operate a clinical service or program and may include but are not limited to the clinical director, discipline chief, and unit or service director); and staff members in a leadership position within the organization.

† **services** Structural divisions of an organization or its staff; also the delivery of care.

‡ "Care" includes individual care, treatment, service, rehabilitation, habilitation, or another program instituted for the individual served by the organization.

4. **Improving performance.** Leadership establishes expectations and plans and manages the performance improvement process. It ensures that processes to design, measure, assess, improve, and maintain the performance of the organization's governance, management, clinical, and support processes are carried out.

Standards

A list of all standards for this function appears below, presented without footnotes or other explanatory text. If you have any questions about a term used here, please refer to the standard as it appears in the next section of this chapter—Standards and Intent Statements.

LD.1 The leaders provide for organizational planning.

LD.1.1 A written plan defines a mission, vision, and values for the organization as well as strategic, operational, program-related, and other plans and policies to achieve them.

LD.1.1.1 Planning addresses all care and services and organizational functions in this manual.

LD.1.1.2 When the organization is part of a multifacility system, its leaders participate in policy decisions that affect the organization.

LD.1.1.3 The organization operates in accordance with applicable laws, rules, and regulations.

LD.1.2 The leaders communicate appropriate information about strategic and other plans throughout the organization.

LD.1.3 The plan(s) includes services to meet individuals' identified needs consistent with the organization's mission.

LD.1.3.1 Services are designed through the collaboration of the organization's leaders with, as appropriate, leaders of the various communities served by the organization and other external organizations.

LD.1.3.2 The design of services is appropriate to the scope and level of care required by individuals served.

LD.1.3.3 Services are designed to be responsive to the needs and expectations of individuals and, as appropriate, their families.

LD.1.3.3.1 The organization gathers, assesses, and takes appropriate action on information that relates to the individual's satisfaction with the care and services provided.

LD.1.3.4 Services are available in a timely manner to meet individuals' needs.

LD.1.3.4.1 Such services are provided either directly or through referral, consultation, or contractual arrangements.

LD.1.3.4.1.1 External sources of services are approved by appropriate leaders.

LD.1.4 The planning process provides a framework for setting performance improvement priorities and identifies how priorities are adjusted in response to unusual or urgent events.

LD.1.5 The leaders develop an annual operating budget and long-term capital expenditure plan in collaboration with representatives from the appropriate disciplines and organizational units, at least as required by applicable law and regulation, including a strategy to monitor the implementation of the plan.

LD.1.5.1 The governing function approves the annual operating budget and long-term capital expenditure plan.

LD.1.5.2 The budget review process considers the appropriateness of the organization's plan for services given the needs of individuals served.

LD.1.5.3 An independent public accountant conducts an annual audit of the organization's financial statements, unless otherwise provided by law.

LD.1.6 Leaders ensure that individuals with the same problems and needs get uniform care throughout the organization.

LD.1.7 The scope of services provided by each program or service of the organization is defined in writing and approved by the organization's leaders.

LD.1.7.1 A written plan guides the provision of services in each program and defines the goals and scope of services offered.

LD.1.7.2 The written plan for services is based on recognized practice standards and guidelines, when available.

LD.1.8 The leaders and appropriate staff participate in the organization's decision-making structures and processes.

LD.1.8.1 Both administrative and clinical leaders have the opportunity to participate in designing and redesigning decision-making processes.

LD.1.8.2 Administrative and clinical leaders collaboratively establish necessary structures, bylaws, rules, regulations, and processes to support clinical activities.

LD.1.8.2.1 Leaders ensure physician input in planning for the provision of medical services.

LD.1.8.2.1.1 In organizations with inpatient programs, the clinical leaders include physician and nursing representation.

LD.1.8.3 Clinical leaders participate in determining the qualifications (training, experience, and documented competence) required for staff assuming specific clinical service responsibilities.

LD.1.9 The leaders develop programs to promote staff recruitment, retention, development, and continuing education.

LD.1.9.1 The leaders develop programs to support staff members' achievement of job-related educational and advancement goals.

LD.2 The leadership of each program or service is effective.

LD.2.1 The leadership of each program or service is responsible for integrating the program or service into the primary functions of the organization.

LD.2.2 The leadership of each program or service is responsible for coordinating and integrating programs and services with other organizational units.

LD.2.3 The leadership of each program or service is responsible for developing and implementing policies and procedures that guide the provision of services.

LD.2.4 The leadership of each program or service is responsible for recommending enough qualified, competent staff to provide care and services.

LD.2.5 The leadership of each program or service is responsible for determining the qualifications and competence of staff who are not independent practitioners and provide care or services.

LD.2.6 The leadership of each program or service is responsible for overseeing continuous assessment and improvement of the quality of care and services.

LD.2.7 The leadership of each program or service is responsible for maintaining applicable quality-control programs.

LD.2.8 The leadership of each program or service is responsible for orientation, in-service training, and continuing education of all persons in the program or service.

LD.2.9 The leadership of each program or service is responsible for recommending space and other resources needed by the program or service.

LD.2.10 The leadership of each program or service is responsible for participating in selection of external sources of services not provided by the program, service, or organization.

LD.2.11 The leadership of each program or service is responsible for ensuring that defined individual rights and responsibilities are honored.

LD.2.12 The leadership of each program or service is responsible for establishing accountability to the governing body.

LD.2.13 The leadership of each program or service is responsible for reviewing and acting on reports and recommendations from committees, programs, and services.

LD.2.14 The leadership of each program or service is responsible for establishing and implementing approved clinical policies.

LD.2.15 The leadership of each program or service is responsible for defining the role of each discipline in clinical care.

LD.2.16 The leadership of each program or service is responsible for verifying the licensure, certification, or registration of the clinical staff, if applicable.

LD.2.17 The leadership of each program or service is responsible for determining the current competence of all clinical staff.

LD.2.18 Leaders organize, direct, and staff services commensurate with the scope of services offered.

LD.2.18.1 Programs or services are directed by one or more individuals whose qualifications, authority, and responsibilities are defined in writing.

LD.2.18.1.1 Responsibility for administrative and clinical direction is defined in writing.

LD.2.18.1.1.1 A qualified professional with appropriate clinical training and experience is responsible for the clinical direction of care and service delivery.

LD.2.18.1.1.2 When there is more than one director of a single program or service, the responsibilities of each are defined in writing.

LD.2.18.1.1.3 When an organization is partially or totally organized on a team or unit basis, the written plan for clinical services delineates the roles and responsibilities of team members in meeting the identified clinical needs of individuals served, consistent with the organization's goals and programs.

LD.3 Services are appropriately integrated throughout the organization.

LD.3.1 The organizational and functional relationships between services are specified in the organization's overall plan for services.

LD.3.2 The leaders foster communication and coordination between individuals and components within the organization.

LD.3.3 The leaders maintain communication with the leaders of corporately or functionally related health care organizations.

LD.3.4 All program or service policies and procedures are developed in collaboration with associated programs or services and approved by the organization's administration and/or clinical staff, as appropriate.

LD.4 The leaders set expectations, develop plans, and manage processes to assess, improve, and maintain the quality of the organization's governance, management, clinical, and support activities.

LD.4.1 The leaders understand performance improvement approaches and methods.

LD.4.2 The leaders adopt an approach to performance improvement that provides for

LD.4.2.1 planning the improvement process;

LD.4.2.2 setting improvement priorities;

LD.4.2.3 systematically assessing performance;

LD.4.2.4 implementing improvement activities based on assessment; and

LD.4.2.5 maintaining achieved improvements.

LD.4.3 The leaders ensure that processes and activities most important to clinical outcomes are continuously and systematically measured, assessed, and improved throughout the organization.

LD.4.3.1 All leaders and managers participate in cross-organizational performance improvement activities, as appropriate to their responsibilities.

LD.4.3.2 Performance improvement information is forwarded to leaders and staff responsible for coordinating organizationwide performance improvement activities.

LD.4.3.3 Responsibility for acting on performance improvement recommendations is assigned and defined in writing.

LD.4.4 The leaders allocate adequate resources for assessment and improvement of the organization's governance, managerial, clinical, and support processes, through

LD.4.4.1 assigning personnel, as needed, to participate in performance improvement activities;

LD.4.4.2 providing adequate time for personnel to participate in performance improvement activities;

LD.4.4.3 creating and maintaining information systems and appropriate data management processes to support collection, management, and analysis of data needed to facilitate ongoing performance improvement; and

LD.4.4.4 providing for personnel training in the approaches to and methods of assessment and improvement.

LD.4.5 The leaders evaluate their effectiveness in improving performance.

Standards and Intent Statements

Organization Planning

Standards

LD.1 *The leaders provide for organizational planning.*

LD.1.1 A written plan defines a mission, vision, and values for the organization as well as strategic, operational, program-related, and other plans and policies to achieve them.

LD.1.1.1 Planning addresses all care and services and organizational functions in this manual.

Intent of LD.1 Through LD.1.1.1

Through planning, the organization's leaders create the framework for providing the organization's behavioral health care services. They develop and carry out an effective planning process that produces timely, well-defined goals. The leaders allocate adequate resources and direct activities to achieve these goals.

Planning is a continuous process that consists of

- developing and communicating a mission that describes the organization's purpose and role in the community;
- revising this mission as necessary;
- assessing the needs of individuals served and other external and internal customers;
- establishing clear long-range, strategic, and operational plans, budgets, resource allocations, and policies;
- eliciting staff input about goals and plans; and
- continuously measuring and assessing performance to ensure that the organization's mission is consistently supported over time.

Standard

LD.1.1.2 When the organization is part of a multifacility system, its leaders participate in policy decisions that affect the organization.

Intent of LD.1.1.2

If the organization is part of a multifacility system, its leaders participate with the appropriate corporate levels of the system in making policy decisions that affect care and service delivery in their organization. Examples of such decisions include adding or eliminating clinical services that would affect the organization's ability to meet the needs of individuals served, or adding or eliminating support services that would affect the staff's ability to provide care to individuals or their families.

The organization clearly describes how its leaders will participate in such decision making. This description can be contained in the organization's or system's organizational plan; a written agreement, letter, memorandum, or description of the leaders' responsibility and authority; meeting minutes documenting the leaders' participation in meetings with corporate levels of the system; or, as appropriate, bylaws, rules, and regulations. The description addresses

- the scope and degree of the leaders' involvement, authority and responsibility in corporate-level policy decisions that affect care and service delivery;
- the means of introducing information from performance improvement activities and other efforts to improve care and services; and
- the process for resolving conflicts between the organization and the overall corporate entity when policy decisions could affect care delivery.

Standard

LD.1.1.3 The organization operates in accordance with applicable laws, rules, and regulations.

Intent of LD.1.1.3

The leaders provide for compliance with applicable federal, state and local law and regulation. The leaders ensure that the organization maintains current licensure or certification by appropriate agencies, as applicable. Other evidence of compliance includes certificates of ownership, articles of incorporation, stock certificates, corporate bylaws and, when applicable, state licensure or certification.

Standard

LD.1.2 The leaders communicate appropriate information about strategic and other plans throughout the organization.

Intent of LD.1.2

The leaders clearly communicate the mission, vision, values, and goals to all members of the organization. An understanding of the mission and goals guides staff in their day-to-day activities, facilitates innovation and motivates staff to follow strategic, operational, program, and other plans. How effectively the leaders communicate the mission may be measured by how well individuals throughout the organization understand it.

For competitive reasons, there may be certain aspects of the strategic plans—and even the vision—that should not become public knowledge. The leaders make reasonable determinations about the information to be communicated. To enhance the organization's effectiveness, the leaders communicate relevant strategic objectives to individuals involved in the organization's daily operations.

Standard

LD.1.3 The plan(s) includes services to meet individuals' identified needs consistent with the organization's mission.

Intent of LD.1.3

Services are designed in response to the needs of populations served, as identified in the planning process. Service planning takes into account

- the population served;
- the organization's mission;
- the scope of services; and
- the care and service delivery needs identified by the direct care staff.

Standard

LD.1.3.1 Services are designed through the collaboration of the organization's leaders with, as appropriate, leaders of the various communities served by the organization and other external organizations.

Intent of LD.1.3.1

Appropriate members of the organization are involved in service planning. Staff who are most knowledgeable about particular services participate in their planning. When planning services in response to an identified community need, every effort is made to involve relevant community leaders and, when appropriate, other provider organizations.

Standard

LD.1.3.2 The design of services is appropriate to the scope and level of care required by individuals served.

Intent of LD.1.3.2

The leaders plan services and care delivery address the behavioral health needs of the population served. Service design is based on the identified needs and conditions of individuals served. Planning establishes processes to ensure that individuals receive care and services that meet their identified needs.

Standards

LD.1.3.3 Services are designed to be responsive to the needs and expectations of individuals and, as appropriate, their families.

LD.1.3.3.1 *The organization gathers, assesses, and takes appropriate action on information that relates to the individual's satisfaction with the care and services provided.*

Intent of LD.1.3.3 and LD.1.3.3.1

The organization measures individuals' involvement in, and satisfaction with, care and services. The leaders incorporate this information into the planning process to improve the quality of care. To do this, the organization

- elicits feedback from individuals served, former individuals served, and families; and
- systematically collects information from individuals served or former individuals served about their satisfaction with specific aspects of the organization's performance.

Feedback can be gathered using satisfaction surveys, phone interviews, follow-up questionnaires, or other methods. This data is then used to assess the satisfaction of individuals served with major clinical care activities and support functions that contribute to the appropriateness, availability, continuity, effectiveness, efficacy, efficiency, respect and caring, safety, and timeliness of services.

Standards

LD.1.3.4 Services are available in a timely manner to meet individuals' needs.

LD.1.3.4.1 Such services are provided either directly or through referral, consultation, or contractual arrangements.

LD.1.3.4.1.1 External sources of services are approved by appropriate leaders.

Intent of LD.1.3.4 Through LD.1.3.4.1.1

As part of the planning process, the organization determines which services it will provide directly to individuals based on their identified needs and in compliance with applicable law and regulation. The organization may decide to provide some services through referral, consultation, or contractual agreement. When services are not provided directly by the organization, a written agreement approved by appropriate leaders describes the services to be provided and requires the source to meet relevant performance expectations of this manual.

Standard

LD.1.4 The planning process provides a framework for setting performance improvement priorities and identifies how priorities are adjusted in response to unusual or urgent events.

Intent of LD.1.4

A framework for setting performance improvement priorities that align with the organization's overall priorities should emerge from the planning process. Planning should also establish a means of reprioritizing performance improvement activities to enable quick response to unusual occurrences or sentinel events.

Standards

LD.1.5 The leaders develop an annual operating budget and long-term capital expenditure plan in collaboration with representatives from the appropriate disciplines and organizational units, at least as required by applicable law and regulation, including a strategy to monitor the implementation of the plan.

LD.1.5.1 The governing function approves the annual operating budget and long-term capital expenditure plan.

LD.1.5.2 The budget review process considers the appropriateness of the organization's plan for services given the needs of individuals served.

Intent of LD.1.5 Through LD.1.5.2

Although these standards do not require an organization to use any particular organizational structure, whatever structure is used should exhibit the following characteristics:

- Leaders include representatives from every appropriate discipline and category of management;
- Leaders are involved in decision-making activities that influence the provision of care, including participating in resource allocation activities to meet the challenges of fiscal pressures and developing the organization's operating budget and long-term capital expenditure planning activities; and
- Leaders participate in meetings, forums, or other occasions when discussion or action focuses on developing or reviewing the following:
  - Strategic plans that affect, involve, or influence care delivery within their particular program or service,
  - Revenue and capital, expense, and personnel budgets that directly or indirectly relate to the staff members' ability to provide care, including the organization's plan for fiscal and other resource allocation,

- ❑ Operational plans that affect staff members' ability to provide appropriate, effective, efficient, efficacious, safe, timely, and continuous care with respect and caring, and
- ❑ Policies that affect staff members and/or the care and services they provide.

The organization's budget describes, in quantifiable terms, the organization's goals and objectives. Since providing care and services is fundamental to the organization's mission, goals, and objectives, the leaders, in collaboration with the appropriate representatives from each program or service, should develop a budget for each program or service. Regardless of the process used or the persons who participate in developing the budget, documentation indicates that the following factors were considered when the department or service-level budget was prepared:

- The assumptions on which the budget is built;
- Use of applicable data and information from the ongoing review of the system for determining the individual's need for care or services, the organization's plan for staffing, assessment and improvement of organizational performance (including risk management and utilization review), and other sources that address how well fiscal and other resource allocations provide for care or services;
- Use of applicable information from the organization's strategic-planning process that indicates any need to refine the fiscal resources allocated for providing care or services; and
- The process used to measure program, service, or other organizational unit performance in relation to the approved budget, including the methods for measuring and acting on identified variances.

Standard

LD.1.5.3 An independent public accountant conducts an annual audit of the organization's financial statements, unless otherwise provided by law.

Intent of LD.1.5.3

A checks-and-balances system is in effect to ensure proper financial management practices. For government programs, this audit is performed in accordance with the regulations of the responsible government agency. The leader's review and approval of the audits is documented.

Standard

LD.1.6 Leaders ensure that individuals with the same problems and needs get uniform care throughout the organization.

Intent of LD.1.6

Individuals with comparable needs should receive the same quality of care or services throughout the organization. The organization's leaders are responsible for ensuring that factors such as different providers or different settings of care do not influence the outcome.

Standards

LD.1.7 The scope of services provided by each program or service of the organization is defined in writing and approved by the organization's leaders.

LD.1.7.1 A written plan guides the provision of services in each program and defines the goals and scope of services offered.

LD.1.7.2 The written plan for services is based on recognized practice standards and guidelines, when available.

Intent of LD.1.7 Through LD.1.7.2

Policies for each program or service describe the kinds of care and services provided by staff to individuals served and their families. The provision of care and services reflects the organization's mission and recognizes the rights of individuals served, the interdependence of care delivery, and organizational ethical issues. Policies and procedures are developed and carried out as required by the population(s) served, the scope and complexity of individuals' need for care, and the knowledge and skill level of the staff members who provide the care delivery. At a minimum, policies and procedures describe how the needs of the individuals served are assessed and met. Recognized practice standards and guidelines are used in planning services.

Standards

LD.1.8 The leaders and appropriate staff participate in the organization's decision-making structures and processes.

LD.1.8.1 Both administrative and clinical leaders have the opportunity to participate in designing and redesigning decision-making processes.

Intent of LD.1.8 and LD.1.8.1

Organization leaders and the directors of appropriate organizational units collaborate in

- developing organizationwide programs, policies, and procedures for assessing and meeting individuals' care and service needs;
- developing and carrying out the organization's plan for care and service delivery;
- participating in the organization's decision-making structures and processes; and
- implementing an effective and ongoing program to measure, assess, and improve the quality of care and services.

Standard

LD.1.8.2 Administrative and clinical leaders collaboratively establish necessary structures, bylaws, rules, regulations, and processes to support clinical activities.

Intent of LD.1.8.2

The intent of this standard is self-evident.

Standard

LD.1.8.2.1 Leaders ensure physician input in planning for the provision of medical services.

Intent of LD.1.8.2.1

Physician participation is essential on issues about individuals' medical needs, including diagnosis, evaluation, and treatment.

Standard

LD.1.8.2.1.1 In organizations with inpatient programs, the clinical leaders include physician and nursing representation.

Intent of LD.1.8.2.1.1

When acute care services are provided, there is participation by a physician and registered nurse in the planning of such services. At a minimum, this includes planning for clinical services, development of clinical policies and procedures, and performance improvement activities.

Standard

LD.1.8.3 Clinical leaders participate in determining the qualifications (training, experience, and documented competence) required for staff assuming specific clinical service responsibilities.

Intent of LD.1.8.3

One of the principal functions of each peer group is to determine the qualifications needed to reach competency in the practice of the discipline, including generic competency (general skills) and special competencies (areas of special competency to carry out specific or specialized interventions). The clinical leaders establish competencies that involve cross-discipline delivery of services. Given these responsibilities, licensure, certification, registration, or demonstration of clinical experience and/or competence comparable to that required for licensure, registration, or certification provides a foundation level to assume specific clinical responsibilities. Other staff members may be assigned to perform specific treatment responsibilities only when supervised by clinical staff qualified by demonstrated licensure, certification, registration, or demonstration of clinical experience and/or competence.

Standards

LD.1.9 The leaders develop programs to promote staff recruitment, retention, development, and continuing education.

LD.1.9.1 The leaders develop programs to support staff members' achievement of job-related educational and advancement goals.

Intent of LD.1.9 and LD.1.9.1

An organization's ability to meet individuals' needs with safe and effective care often depends on attracting and keeping adequate numbers and types of qualified, competent staff. When developing staff recruitment, retention, development, and continuing education programs, the leaders consider the following factors:

- The organization's mission;
- The populations served by the organization, service, or program, and the degree and complexity of care and services required by these individuals and their families;
- The technology used in the delivery of care and services;
- The type and degree of care and services expected by the organization, clinical staff, individuals, and families;
- Staff members' identified learning needs;
- Processes for recognizing the expertise and performance of staff members providing care and services; and

- Issues identified by staff members as influencing their decisions to continue employment with the organization.

Because retention activities provide more long-term benefit than recruitment, the leaders support staff members' educational and advancement goals that contribute to the organization's mission. The leaders collaboratively develop and carry out programs to help staff achieve these goals.

Whenever possible, staff members should be encouraged to participate in appropriate professional associations and continuing educational activities outside the organization.

Directing Services

Standard

LD.2 *The leadership of each program or service is effective.*

Intent of LD.2

Effective leadership at the program or service level is also important to achieving the organization's mission and goals. Much like organization-level leaders, program or service leaders play a critical role in creating an environment that enables the organization to meet or exceed its goals. Embracing the same leadership qualities evident at the organizationwide level, these leaders are effective communicators who clearly articulate the organization's mission to all members of their program or service. It is their responsibility to operationalize the organization's mission and goals within the program or service.

Program or service leaders support staff and encourage them to take responsibility for work processes. The leaders foster a sense of ownership and accountability for work and motivate staff to continuously improve their performance, thereby improving the organization's performance.

Standards

LD.2.1 The leadership of each program or service is responsible for integrating the program or service into the primary functions of the organization.

LD.2.2 The leadership of each program or service is responsible for coordinating and integrating programs and services with other organizational units.

LD.2.3 The leadership of each program or service is responsible for developing and implementing policies and procedures that guide the provision of services.

LD.2.4 The leadership of each program or service is responsible for recommending enough qualified, competent staff to provide care and services.

LD.2.5 The leadership of each program or service is responsible for determining the qualifications and competence of staff who are not independent practitioners and provide care or services.

LD.2.6 The leadership of each program or service is responsible for overseeing continuous assessment and improvement of the quality of care and services.

LD.2.7 The leadership of each program or service is responsible for maintaining applicable quality-control programs.

LD.2.8 The leadership of each program or service is responsible for orientation, in-service training, and continuing education of all persons in the program or service.

LD.2.9 The leadership of each program or service is responsible for recommending space and other resources needed by the program or service.

LD.2.10 The leadership of each program or service is responsible for participating in selection of external sources of services not provided by the program, service, or organization.

LD.2.11 The leadership of each program or service is responsible for ensuring that defined individual rights and responsibilities are honored.

LD.2.12 The leadership of each program or service is responsible for establishing accountability to the governing body.

LD.2.13 The leadership of each program or service is responsible for reviewing and acting on reports and recommendations from committees, programs, and services.

LD.2.14 The leadership of each program or service is responsible for establishing and implementing approved clinical policies.

LD.2.15 The leadership of each program or service is responsible for defining the role of each discipline in clinical care.

LD.2.16 The leadership of each program or service is responsible for verifying the licensure, certification, or registration of the clinical staff, if applicable.

LD.2.17 The leadership of each program or service is responsible for determining the current competence of all clinical staff.

Intent of LD.2.1 Through LD.2.17

The leaders of each program or service are responsible for its ongoing, effective operation and for the continuous assessment and improvement of its performance. In addition to overseeing internal functioning, program or service leaders are responsible for

- integrating the program or service into the overall functioning of the organization;
- coordinating services with other programs within the organization; and
- continuously improving the services provided by the program or service.

Program or service leaders ensure that their staff's learning needs are identified and addressed at appropriate and timely intervals. Program or service leaders provide continuing education either directly or by giving staff time to attend other educational programs within or outside the organization. Leaders or their designees collaborate with others responsible for organization-wide education on such topics as infection control, safety management, life safety, emergency preparedness, cardiopulmonary resuscitation, and other emergency procedures and techniques.

When outside service providers are selected, the leaders of relevant programs or services participate in assessing available options and making recommendations.

Standard

LD.2.18 *Leaders organize, direct, and staff services commensurate with the scope of services offered.*

Intent of LD.2.18

The leaders establish, through the chief executive officer, a comprehensive policy framework for directing the organization's operations and services and providing enough resources to accomplish the organization's mission, philosophy, goals, and objectives. Allocation of resources is directly related to the identified needs of the organization's age and disability groups and the requirements of the treatment setting. Resource needs and types are determined by the scope of services provided.

Standards

LD.2.18.1 Programs or services are directed by one or more individuals whose qualifications, authority, and responsibilities are defined in writing.

LD.2.18.1.1 Responsibility for administrative and clinical direction is defined in writing.

LD.2.18.1.1.1 A qualified professional with appropriate clinical training and experience is responsible for the clinical direction of care and service delivery.

LD.2.18.1.1.2 When there is more than one director of a single program or service, the responsibilities of each are defined in writing.

LD.2.18.1.1.3 When an organization is partially or totally organized on a team or unit basis, the written plan for clinical services delineates the roles and responsibilities of team members in meeting the identified clinical needs of individuals served, consistent with the organization's goals and programs.

Intent of LD.2.18.1 Through LD.2.18.1.1.3

Programs and services may be directed by a qualified professional with appropriate training and experience or by a qualified licensed independent practitioner who has appropriate clinical privileges. If the director is not a clinician, then another qualified individual is responsible for directing clinical services.

The directors of programs and services also have adequate management skills to effectively direct the programs or services and fulfill their many responsibilities. Some of these responsibilities may be delegated to others in the program, service, or organization. It may be appropriate for the program or service director to delegate some responsibilities for policies and procedures, technical staffing, equipment and space, quality control programs, safety, or performance improvement activities to others who are more qualified to address them. Nonetheless, the director has ultimate responsibility for the activities in LD.2.1 through LD.2.17.

When there is more than one director of a program or service, the responsibilities of each are defined in writing to facilitate collaboration, cooperation, and resolution of decision-making conflicts.

Treatment roles and responsibilities of team members are consistent with the needs of individuals served and the service's goals and objectives. Assignment of staff roles and responsibilities may vary based on the needs of the organization's age and disability groups.

Integrating Services

Standards

LD.3 *Services are appropriately integrated throughout the organization.*

LD.3.1 The organizational and functional relationships between services are specified in the organization's overall plan for services.

LD.3.2 The leaders foster communication and coordination between individuals and components within the organization.

LD.3.3 The leaders maintain communication with the leaders of corporately- or functionally-related health care organizations.

LD.3.4 All program or service policies and procedures are developed in collaboration with associated programs or services and approved by the organization's administration and/or clinical staff, as appropriate.

Intent of LD.3 Through LD.3.4

Integrating each program or service into the overall functioning of the organization is one of the primary responsibilities of the organization's leaders and program or service directors. Service integration is accomplished through

- joint planning and policy development;
- an explicit organizational structure; and
- good communication.

Role in Improving Performance

Standard

LD.4 The leaders set expectations, develop plans, and manage processes to assess, improve, and maintain the quality of the organization's governance, management, clinical, and support activities.

Intent of LD.4

The role of the organization's leaders is paramount to the success of organizationwide efforts to improve performance. When operating effectively, the organization's leadership guides the organization to achieve new heights in performance. For many organizations, maintaining performance levels will be equally important.

Standard

LD.4.1 The leaders understand performance improvement approaches and methods.

Intent of LD.4.1

For performance improvement efforts to be successful, the leaders must understand performance improvement principles, methods, and practices. The leaders are educated in performance improvement so that they can effectively direct and carry out performance improvement activities.

Standards

LD.4.2 *The leaders adopt an approach to performance improvement that provides for*

LD.4.2.1 planning the improvement process;

LD.4.2.2 setting improvement priorities;

LD.4.2.3 systematically assessing performance;

LD.4.2.4 implementing improvement activities based on assessment; and

LD.4.2.5 maintaining achieved improvements.

Intent of LD.4.2 Through LD.4.2.5

The leaders select an approach to performance improvement that clearly defines how all levels of the organization will address improvement issues. The leaders communicate this approach throughout the organization and lead the effort to implement it.

Performance improvement activities are collaborative and interdisciplinary. All appropriate individuals and professionals work together to plan and implement them.

There are many valid performance improvement methodologies. Although the approach selected must incorporate the essential processes described in the standards, it will reflect the organization's leadership style.

Standard

LD.4.3 The leaders ensure that processes and activities most important to clinical outcomes are continuously and systematically measured, assessed, and improved throughout the organization.

Intent of LD.4.3

The leaders set performance improvement priorities and actively promote effective measurement, assessment, and improvement of performance. They focus the organization's efforts on improving care-delivery processes, especially those that are essential to providing consistent quality of care throughout the organization.

Each relevant program or service participates in organizationwide performance measurement, assessment, and improvement activities.*

---

* As described in the "Improving Organization Performance" chapter of this manual.

Standard

LD.4.3.1 All leaders and managers participate in cross-organizational performance improvement activities, as appropriate to their responsibilities.

Intent of LD.4.3.1

Leaders and directors must engage all staff with managerial responsibilities in the process of performance improvement. This requires establishing clear communication processes and assigning accountability for follow-through.

Leading by example is important. Leaders set the tone for participation in interdisciplinary performance improvement activities by participating in such activities themselves. Because performance improvement is not a process that can be delegated to nonmanagement staff alone, all leaders are responsible for team building. Cross-organizational performance improvement activities are less effective when only nonmanagement staff are involved.

Standard

LD.4.3.2 Performance improvement information is forwarded to leaders and staff responsible for coordinating organizationwide performance improvement activities.

Intent of LD.4.3.2

A successful, coordinated performance improvement process depends on communicating its conclusions and recommendations to individuals responsible for carrying out and coordinating improvements. Accountability is established for specific improvements to motivate their implementation. To do this, leaders also need relevant information from performance improvement activities.

Standard

LD.4.3.3 Responsibility for acting on performance improvement recommendations is assigned and defined in writing.

Intent of LD.4.3.3

For process and procedure improvements to be done successfully, accountabilities must be defined and follow-up action taken. Follow-up action begins with a document that assigns responsibility for acting on performance improvement recommendations to individuals, programs, or other services. The document clearly describes the action to be taken, time frames, and other assignment parameters.

Standards

LD.4.4 *The leaders allocate adequate resources for assessment and improvement of the organization's governance, managerial, clinical, and support processes, through*

LD.4.4.1 assigning personnel, as needed, to participate in performance improvement activities;

LD.4.4.2 providing adequate time for personnel to participate in performance improvement activities;

LD.4.4.3 creating and maintaining information systems and appropriate data management processes to support collection, management, and analysis of data needed to facilitate ongoing performance improvement; and

LD.4.4.4 providing for personnel training in the approaches to and methods of assessment and improvement.

Intent of LD.4.4 Through LD.4.4.4

Effective performance improvement cannot be achieved without allocation of essential human, technical, and financial resources. Staff involved in improvement activities should know how to find resources and training needed to successfully contribute to improvement.

Standard

LD.4.5 The leaders evaluate their effectiveness in improving performance.

Intent of LD.4.5

Effective leadership is essential to carrying out and maintaining an improvement program. The performance improvement framework in the "Improving Organization Performance" chapter of this manual is used to design, measure, assess, and improve the organization's performance of the leadership function, as well as the leaders' contribution to performance improvement.

The leaders

- set measurable objectives for their work to improve organization performance;
- gather information to assess their effectiveness in improving performance;
- use pre-established, objective process criteria to analyze and assess their effectiveness;
- draw conclusions about their contribution to performance improvement;
- develop and implement improvements in their activities; and
- evaluate the effectiveness of improvements to their activities.

Management of the Environment of Care

Overview

The environment of care is a crucial factor in providing care and achieving good outcomes. The **goal** of this function* is to provide a safe, accessible, effective, and efficient environment for individuals served, staff members, and others in the organization. Achieving this goal depends on performing the following processes:

- Planning by organization leaders for the space, equipment, and resources needed to safely and effectively support the services provided. Planning and design are consistent with the organization's mission, vision, and values.
- Educating staff about the role of the environment in safely and effectively supporting care. The organization educates staff about physical characteristics and processes for environmental monitoring and reporting.
- Developing performance standards to measure staff and organization performance in managing and improving the environment of care.
- Carrying out plans to create and manage the organization's environment of care. An Information Collection and Evaluation System (ICES) is developed and used to continuously measure, assess, and improve the status of the environment of care.†

Effective management of the environment of care includes processes and activities to

- reduce and control environmental hazards and risks;
- prevent accidents and injuries; and
- maintain safe conditions for individuals served, visitors, and staff.

The standards in this chapter focus on how everyone in the organization participates in the processes and activities that make the environment of care safe and effective. They also address appropriate leaders' responsibility for identifying and communicating environment of care needs and allocating appropriate space, equipment, and resources to safely and effectively support the organization's services.

Note 1: *The standards in this chapter do not prescribe any particular structure (such as a formal safety committee), job description (such as a safety officer), or format for the required designs and planning activities.*

Note 2: *The standards do not require the Statement of Conditions™ to be completed by anyone other than an employee of the organization. This Statement of Conditions™ is used as the basis for corrective actions needed to make the environment of care as safe and useful as possible for staff and individuals served.*

---

* **function** A goal-directed, inter-related series of processes.

† **environment of care** A variety of sites where behavioral health care or services are provided. Such environments have three basic components: the buildings, equipment, and people.

Standards

A list of all standards for this function appears below, presented without footnotes or other explanatory text. If you have any questions about a term used here, please refer to the standard as it appears in the next section of this chapter—Standards and Intent Statements.

EC.1 The organization establishes an environment of care that meets the needs of individuals served, encourages a positive self-image, and respects their human dignity.

EC.1.1 Waiting or reception areas are comfortable; their design, location, and furnishings accommodate visitors and individuals served, the anticipated waiting time, the need for privacy and/or support from staff, and the organization's goals.

EC.1.2 Enough restrooms are available for the number of individuals served.

EC.1.3 The design, structure, furnishing, and lighting of the environment promote clear visual perceptions of people and functions.

EC.1.3.1 Lighting is controlled by individuals served, when appropriate.

EC.1.3.2 The environment offers views of the outdoors, where possible.

EC.1.3.3 Mirrors that distort as little as possible are placed at reasonable heights in appropriate places to aid in grooming and enhance the self-awareness of individuals served.

EC.1.3.4 The environment minimizes distractions that interfere with therapeutic activities.

EC.1.3.5 The environment maximizes the individual's involvement in leisure activities.

EC.1.4 The organization promotes awareness of time and season.

EC.1.5 A telephone is available for private conversations.

EC.1.6 Ventilation contributes to the environment's habitability.

EC.1.6.1 All areas and surfaces are free of undesirable odors.

EC.1.7 Furnishings and equipment suitable to the population served are available.

EC.1.8 Structural restraints are used in accordance with the organization's mission and program goals.

EC.1.9 Dining areas are comfortable, attractive, and pleasant.

EC.1.9.1 Meals and snacks are served at times that are normal and appropriate for the ages of the individuals served.

EC.1.9.2 Depending on program goals, facilities are available for serving snacks, preparing meals for special occasions, and engaging in recreational activities.

EC.1.9.3 The facilities for serving snacks, preparing meals, and engaging in recreational activities support participation by the individuals served.

EC.1.10 The dining rooms are adequately supervised.

EC.1.10.1 Staff are available to help individuals when needed.

EC.1.10.2 Each individual served gets an adequate amount and variety of food.

EC.1.11 The organization ensures privacy for individuals served.

EC.1.11.1 Sleeping rooms have doors for privacy.

EC.1.11.2 In rooms having more than one individual, privacy is provided for dressing.

EC.1.11.3 In rooms having from four to eight individuals, privacy is provided by partitioning or furniture placement.

EC.1.11.4 Except when clinically justified in writing, based on program requirements, no more than eight individuals sleep in a room.

EC.1.11.5 Sleeping areas are assigned based on individual need for group support, privacy, or independence.

EC.1.12 In accordance with the needs of the individuals served, good standards of personal hygiene and grooming are taught and maintained, particularly in regard to bathing, brushing teeth, caring for hair and nails, and using the toilet, with due regard for privacy.

EC.1.12.1 Individuals served get the help needed to perform these activities and, when indicated, assume responsibility for self-care.

EC.1.12.2 Incontinent individuals are cleaned or bathed immediately after voiding or soiling, with due regard for privacy.

EC.1.12.3 When appropriate to the service setting and length of stay, individuals served have access to the services of a barber or beautician, either in the organization or community.

EC.1.12.4 Articles for grooming and personal hygiene appropriate to the individual's age, developmental level, and clinical status are readily available in a space reserved near the individual's sleeping area.

EC.1.13 Closet and drawer space are provided for storing individuals' personal property and items for personal use.

EC.1.13.1 If clinically indicated, an individual's personal articles may be kept under lock and key by staff.

EC.1.14 Individuals served are allowed to keep and display appropriate personal belongings and add suitable personal touches to their surroundings.

EC.1.15 Individuals served are encouraged to take responsibility for maintaining their own living quarters and for day-to-day housekeeping activities of the program, as appropriate to their clinical status.

EC.1.16 Individuals served wear suitable clothing.

EC.1.17 The organization has a policy on the availability and care of pets and other animals.

EC.1.18 Unless contraindicated for therapeutic reasons, the organization accommodates the needs of individuals to be outdoors.

EC.2 The organization designs a safe, accessible, effective, and efficient environment consistent with its mission, services, and law and regulation.

EC.2.1 A management plan addresses safety.

EC.2.2 A management plan addresses security.

EC.2.3 A management plan addresses control of hazardous materials and wastes.

EC.2.4 A management plan addresses emergency preparedness.

EC.2.5 A management plan addresses life safety.

EC.2.5.1 Management activities temporarily compensate for life-safety deficiencies and construction hazards.

EC.2.5.2 The environment is designed and maintained to comply with the *Life Safety Code.*®

EC.2.6 A management plan addresses medical equipment.

EC.2.7 A management plan addresses utility systems.

EC.2.8 A management plan addresses the physical environment.

EC.2.8.1 When designing the environment, the organization uses design criteria from the health care community.

EC.2.8.2 The organization has enough space and equipment for staff to provide the services offered.

EC.2.8.3 A policy prohibiting smoking is developed.

EC.2.9 An organizationwide Information Collection and Evaluation System is developed.

EC.3 The organization provides a safe, accessible, effective, and efficient environment consistent with its mission, services, and law and regulation through training, drills, performance, and maintenance.

EC.3.1 The management plans are carried out.

EC.3.1.1 Staff have been oriented to and educated about the environment and have the knowledge and skills to perform their responsibilities under the management plans.

EC.3.1.2 Emergency drills are conducted regularly.

EC.3.1.3 The operational components of the management plans are maintained, tested, and inspected.

EC.3.2 An organizationwide Information Collection and Evaluation System is used to monitor performance data and known risk factors to identify environment of care safety management issues and make recommendations for resolving these.

Standards and Intent Statements

Therapeutic Environment

Standards

EC.1 *The organization establishes an environment of care that meets the needs of individuals served, encourages a positive self-image, and respects their human dignity.*

EC.1.1 Waiting or reception areas are comfortable; their design, location, and furnishings accommodate visitors and individuals served, the anticipated waiting time, the need for privacy and/or support from staff, and the organization's goals.

EC.1.2 Enough restrooms are available for the number of individuals served.

Intent of EC.1 Through EC.1.2

The buildings and grounds should promote a therapeutic environment that enhances the self-image of individuals served. The physical structure, grounds, and space are adequate to meet the needs of individuals served and their families and contribute to the enhancement of the organization's neighborhood and community.

Available outdoor space is adequate, based on programs offered and the needs, age, and disability of individuals served. Physically challenged people have access to all necessary services and programs in accordance with the Americans with Disabilities Act (ADA); in federally owned and operated facilities, physically challenged people have access to all necessary services and programs in accordance with the Uniform Federal Accessibility Standards (UFAS).

Waiting and reception areas are adequate in size and number and staffed according to the needs of individuals served. Enough restrooms are available for the persons using the facility. Drinking fountains or water coolers are available and appropriate for the age and disability groups served (for example, children or wheelchair-bound individuals). Only single-use disposable cups are used, if necessary.

Standards

EC.1.3 The design, structure, furnishing, and lighting of the environment promote clear visual perceptions of people and functions.

EC.1.3.1 Lighting is controlled by individuals served, when appropriate.

EC.1.3.2 The environment offers views of the outdoors, where possible.

EC.1.3.3 Mirrors that distort as little as possible are placed at reasonable heights in appropriate places to aid in grooming and enhance the self-awareness of individuals served.

EC.1.3.4 The environment minimizes distractions that interfere with therapeutic activities.

EC.1.3.5 The environment maximizes the individual's involvement in leisure activities.

EC.1.4 The organization promotes awareness of time and season.

EC.1.5 A telephone is available for private conversations.

EC.1.6 Ventilation contributes to the environment's habitability.

EC.1.6.1 All areas and surfaces are free of undesirable odors.

EC.1.7 Furnishings and equipment suitable to the population served are available.

Intent of EC.1.3 Through EC.1.7

The organization provides indoor and outdoor environments that support an individual's dignity. Lighting is appropriate and, when possible, controlled by the individuals served. Outdoor views should be enhanced by windows or skylights. Mirrors cause minimal distortion, are located in grooming areas, and are hung at appropriate heights. Use and location of noise-producing equipment and appliances, such as televisions, radios, and stereos, do not interfere with other therapeutic activities. Furnishings and equipment are in good repair, and all areas are attractively decorated. When furnishings and equipment break, they are repaired promptly.

The organization encourages interaction between staff and individuals served. Therapeutic programs should provide recreational and leisure-time activities, and the equipment to perform these functions should be kept in good working order. Space and equipment are available for table games and hobbies. Toys, games, and arts and crafts supplies and equipment are available. Books, magazines, and newspapers are current.

Clocks and calendars are available in major use areas such as day rooms, recreational areas, and individuals' rooms, if appropriate. Telephones are available for private conversations and accessible to physically challenged individuals. There is adequate ventilation to remove odors and provide direct outside air to each individual's room through air-conditioning or working windows.

Standard

EC.1.8 Structural restraints are used in accordance with the organization's mission and program goals.

Intent of EC.1.8

a. Structural restraints (for example, fences, door-locking devices) are used consistent with the individual's needs, program policy, law, and regulation to provide the least restrictive environment.
b. Emergency access provisions are provided to all locked occupied spaces.
c. Review and approval of the use of structural restraints by the organization's leaders is documented. Consideration should be given to the safety, rights, and security of the individual when approving the use of structural restraints.

Standards

EC.1.9 Dining areas are comfortable, attractive, and pleasant.

EC.1.9.1 Meals and snacks are served at times that are normal and appropriate for the ages of the individuals served.

EC.1.9.2 Depending on program goals, facilities are available for serving snacks, preparing meals for special occasions, and engaging in recreational activities.

EC.1.9.3 The facilities for serving snacks, preparing meals, and engaging in recreational activities support participation by the individuals served.

Intent of EC.1.9 Through EC.1.9.3

Dining areas are designed to promote social interaction, and the timing of meals and snacks promotes commonly recognized daily routines. Consistent with its mission, the organization has program areas and equipment available for serving snacks, preparing meals for special occasions, and having picnics or other recreational activities.

Standards

EC.1.10 The dining rooms are adequately supervised.

EC.1.10.1 Staff are available to help individuals when needed.

EC.1.10.2 Each individual served gets an adequate amount and variety of food.

Intent of EC.1.10 Through EC.1.10.2

Dining areas are arranged to seat small groups, and staff members are assigned to offer supervision and assistance if needed.

Standards

EC.1.11 *The organization ensures privacy for individuals served.*

EC.1.11.1 Sleeping rooms have doors for privacy.

EC.1.11.2 In rooms having more than one individual, privacy is provided for dressing.

EC.1.11.3 In rooms having from four to eight individuals, privacy is provided by partitioning or furniture placement.

EC.1.11.4 Except when clinically justified in writing, based on program requirements, no more than eight individuals sleep in a room.

EC.1.11.5 Sleeping areas are assigned based on individual need for group support, privacy, or independence.

Intent of EC.1.11 Through EC.1.11.5

The number of individuals in a room is appropriate to the organization's goals and to the ages, developmental levels, and clinical needs of individuals served. Staff respect the right to privacy by knocking on the door of an individual's room before entering. Sleeping rooms have doors for privacy that are removed only when justified for sound clinical reasons. In rooms having more than one individual, privacy is provided for dressing. Unless clinically justified in writing, no more than eight individuals should be sleeping in a room. Individuals who need extra sleep or greater privacy are assigned to bedrooms where no more than two persons sleep.

Standards

EC.1.12 In accordance with the needs of the individuals served, good standards of personal hygiene and grooming are taught and maintained, particularly in regard to bathing, brushing teeth, caring for hair and nails, and using the toilet, with due regard for privacy.

EC.1.12.1 Individuals served get the help needed to perform these activities and, when indicated, assume responsibility for self-care.

EC.1.12.2 Incontinent individuals are cleaned or bathed immediately after voiding or soiling, with due regard for privacy.

EC.1.12.3 When appropriate to the service setting and length of stay, individuals served have access to the services of a barber or beautician, either in the organization or community.

EC.1.12.4 Articles for grooming and personal hygiene appropriate to the individual's age, developmental level, and clinical status are readily available in a space reserved near the individual's sleeping area.

Intent of EC.1.12 Through EC.1.12.4

Personal hygiene areas provide privacy. Bathrooms and toilets have partitions and doors; toilets have seats. Bedroom areas have space for individuals' grooming and personal hygiene articles; shelves, closets, and drawer space are provided. Incontinent individuals are kept clean and dry after soiling and are given appropriate privacy.

As appropriate, staff supervise the implementation of standards of care for personal hygiene (for example, grooming, oral hygiene, foot care, hair and nail care) and review them; the supervision and review is documented in individual schedules and clinical records. Individuals are evaluated for self-care capabilities. The organization offers education and grooming activities based on each individual's needs.

Standards

EC.1.13 Closet and drawer space are provided for storing individuals' personal property and items for personal use.

EC.1.13.1 If clinically indicated, an individual's personal articles may be kept under lock and key by staff.

Intent of EC.1.13 and EC.1.13.1

Space is provided for personal property to help ensure privacy. Locked storage space is available for those requesting it. Individuals served are informed when articles for grooming or other uses reconsidered dangerous and thus contraindicated. Such restrictions and their clinical rationale are documented in the clinical record.

Standard

EC.1.14 Individuals served are allowed to keep and display appropriate personal belongings and add suitable personal touches to their surroundings.

Intent of EC.1.14

Individuals served are allowed to keep and display personal belongings and to add other suitable personal touches to their surroundings. The organization has written rules to govern personal displays and supplies the necessary equipment (such as bulletin boards) to allow this. When restrictions in use of personal belongings are incorporated into a privilege program, they must be noted in an individual's behavior-management plan or program protocol and documented in the individual's treatment plan.

Standard

EC.1.15 Individuals served are encouraged to take responsibility for maintaining their own living quarters and for day-to-day housekeeping activities of the program, as appropriate to their clinical status.

Intent of EC.1.15

The individuals served maintain their own living quarters and take responsibility for day-to-day housekeeping activities in a manner commensurate with their age and disability group. These activities are addressed in orientation programs.

Standard

EC.1.16 Individuals served wear suitable clothing.

Intent of EC.1.16

Individuals served are allowed to wear their own clothing as part of the normalization process. If the organization supplies clothing, it is individualized and personalized for and by the individuals served. Clothing provided by the program is appropriate, durable, suitable to the season, and similar to that worn by persons in the external environment. Enough clothing is made available to permit laundering, cleaning, and repair.

Standard

EC.1.17 The organization has a policy on the availability and care of pets and other animals.

Intent of EC.1.17

If the organization allows pets, it must have policies on their care consistent with the organization's goals and good health and sanitation requirements. These policies must also be consistent with standards in the "Surveillance, Prevention, and Control of Infection" chapter of this manual (page 257).

Standard

EC.1.18 Unless contraindicated for therapeutic reasons, the organization accommodates the needs of individuals to be outdoors.

Intent of EC.1.18

Therapeutic programs provide for recreational and leisure-time activities. Equipment used in these activities is kept in good working order. The organization arranges for activities in nearby parks, playgrounds, countryside, and on the organization's grounds.

Design

Standard

EC.2 *The organization designs a safe, accessible, effective, and efficient environment consistent with its mission, services, and law and regulation.*

Intent of EC.2

The organization designs its environment based on management processes. These processes include safety, security, control of hazardous materials and waste, emergency preparedness, life safety, medical equipment, and utilities systems. Performance improvement activities include setting performance standards for assessing staff knowledge and skills as well as systems and equipment.

Standard

EC.2.1 A management plan addresses safety.

Intent of EC.2.1

A plan describes how the organization establishes and maintains a safety-management program to protect individuals served, staff, and visitors from injury. The plan provides processes for

a. conducting risk assessments that proactively evaluate the impact of buildings, grounds, equipment,* occupants, and internal physical systems on safety;
b. examining safety issues by appropriate representatives;
c. reporting and investigating all incidents of property damage, occupational illness, and injury to the individuals served, staff, or visitors;
d. conducting ongoing hazard surveillance, including response to product safety recalls;
e. appointing a qualified individual(s) to address safety issues and oversee development, implementation, and monitoring of safety management;
f. identifying an individual(s) to intervene whenever conditions pose an immediate threat to life or health or threaten damage to equipment or buildings;
g. an orientation and education program;
h. ongoing monitoring of performance regarding actual or potential risks related to one or more of the following:
   - Staff knowledge and skills
   - Level of staff participation
   - Monitoring and inspection activities
   - Emergency and incident reporting

* "Nonmedical equipment" includes, but is not limited to, art and music therapy supplies, books, sports equipment, pool chlorine dispensers, food preparation or laundry equipment, and personal care equipment such as hair dryers and nail clippers.

- Inspection, preventive maintenance, and testing of equipment;

i. distributing, practicing, enforcing, and reviewing safety policies and procedures as often as needed; and
j. evaluating the safety-management plan annually.

Standard

EC.2.2 A management plan addresses security.

Intent of EC.2.2

A plan describes how the organization establishes and maintains a security management program to protect individuals served, staff, and visitors from harm. The plan provides processes for

a. leaders' designation of staff responsible for developing, implementing, and monitoring the security management plan;
b. addressing security issues concerning individuals served, visitors, staff, and property;
c. reporting and investigating all security incidents involving individuals served, visitors, staff, or property;
d. providing identification, when appropriate, for all staff, individuals served, or visitors;
e. controlling access to sensitive areas, as determined by the organization;
f. an orientation and education program addressing security management;
g. ongoing monitoring of performance regarding actual or potential risks related to one or more of the following:
   - Staff knowledge and skills
   - Level of staff participation
   - Monitoring and inspection activities
   - Emergency and incident reporting
   - Inspection, preventive maintenance, and testing of equipment;
h. emergency procedures that address security incidents or failures; and
i. evaluating the security management plan annually.

Standard

EC.2.3 A management plan addresses control of hazardous materials and wastes*.

Intent of EC.2.3

A plan describes how the organization establishes and maintains a program to safely control hazardous materials and wastes. The plan provides processes for

a. selecting, handling, storing, using, and disposing of hazardous materials and wastes from receipt or generation through use or final disposal;

---

* **hazardous materials and wastes** Materials, the handling, use, and storage of which are guided by local, state, or federal regulation (for example, the Occupational Safety and Health Administration's (OSHA's) Regulations for Bloodborne Pathogens regarding the disposal of blood and blood-soaked items; Nuclear Regulatory Commission's regulations for the handling and disposal of radioactive waste), and hazardous energy sources (for example, ionizing or nonionizing radiation, lasers, microwave, or ultrasound).

The Joint Commission recognizes that definitions of hazardous waste differ. At this time, federal regulations do not define infectious waste or medical waste as hazardous waste. However, the intent of this standard is to implement a management process that includes all materials and wastes that require special handling to minimize occupational and environmental hazards. Infectious waste and medical waste fall into the special handling category because of recognized occupational exposure issues that must be addressed.

b. establishing written criteria in accordance with applicable law and regulation to identify, evaluate, and inventory hazardous materials and wastes used or generated;
c. managing chemical wastes, chemotherapeutic wastes, radioactive wastes, and regulated medical or infectious wastes, including sharps;
d. monitoring and disposing of hazardous gases and vapors;
e. providing adequate and appropriate space and equipment for safe handling and storage of hazardous materials and wastes;
f. reporting and investigating all hazardous materials or waste spills, exposures, and other incidents;
g. an orientation and education program addressing control of hazardous materials and wastes;
h. ongoing monitoring of performance regarding actual or potential risks related to one or more of the following:
   - Staff knowledge and skills
   - Level of staff participation
   - Monitoring and inspection activities
   - Emergency and incident reporting
   - Inspection, preventive maintenance, and testing of equipment;
i. emergency procedures that describe the specific precautions, procedures, and protective equipment used during hazardous material and waste spills or exposures; and
j. evaluating the hazardous materials and waste management plan annually.

Standard

EC.2.4 A management plan addresses emergency preparedness.

Intent of EC.2.4

A plan describes how the organization establishes and maintains an emergency-preparedness management program to ensure effective response to disasters* or emergencies affecting the operations of the organization. The plan provides processes for

a. carrying out specific procedures in response to a variety of disasters or emergencies;
b. defining and, when appropriate, integrating the organization's role with communitywide emergency-preparedness efforts;
c. notifying external authorities of emergencies;
d. notifying staff when emergency response measures are initiated;
e. assigning available staff in emergencies to cover all necessary staff positions;
f. managing space and supplies;
g. providing for back-up services if necessary;
h. a back-up communication system in the event of failure during disasters and emergencies;
i. an orientation and education program for staff who participate in the emergency preparedness plan;
j. ongoing monitoring of performance regarding actual or potential risks related to one or more of the following:
   - Staff knowledge and skills
   - Level of staff participation

---

* **disasters** Natural or man-made events that significantly disrupt the environment, such as damage to the organization's buildings and grounds due to severe wind storms, tornadoes, hurricanes, or earthquakes. Also, events which disrupt care and treatment, such as loss of utilities (power, water, and telephones) due to floods, riots, accidents, or emergencies within the organization or in the surrounding community.

- Monitoring and inspection activities
- Emergency and incident reporting
- Inspection, preventive maintenance, and testing of equipment;

k. evaluating the emergency-preparedness management plan annually.

Standard

EC.2.5 A management plan addresses life safety.

Intent of EC.2.5

A plan describes how the organization establishes and maintains a life safety management program* to provide a fire-safe environment. The plan provides processes for

a. protecting individuals served, staff, visitors, and property from fire, smoke, and other products of combustion;

   Note 1: *The following must be provided for*
   - *all therapeutic foster care homes, and*
   - *all buildings (owned, operated, or leased by the organization) housing three or less individuals served:*
     - *Emergency procedures to respond to fire (including identifying primary and secondary means of escape features);*
     - *A door into the sleeping room of the individual served;*
     - *From the sleeping room of the individual served:*
       - *an operable exterior window large enough for emergency escape or*
       - *a door leading directly to the outside, or*
       - *access to a second and remote means of escape; and*
     - *A smoke detector in the sleeping room of the individual served.*

   Note 2: *In buildings (owned, operated, or leased by the organization) housing more than three individuals served, the building must comply with standard EC.2.5.2.*

b. inspecting, testing, and maintaining fire protection and life safety equipment and components on a regular basis in accordance with standard EC.3.1.3;

c. communicating fire protection deficiencies, failures, and user errors to the appointed individual or, if one exists, the safety committee;

d. an orientation and education program addressing life safety;

e. ongoing monitoring of performance regarding actual or potential risks related to one or more of the following:
   - Staff knowledge and skills
   - Level of staff participation
   - Monitoring and inspection activities
   - Emergency and incident reporting
   - Inspection, preventive maintenance, and testing of equipment;

f. emergency procedures that address life safety incidents; and

g. evaluating the life safety management plan annually.

---

* **life safety management program** The organization's documented management plan describing processes for protecting individuals served, staff, visitors, and property from fire and the products of combustion (smoke) and maintaining all structural features of fire protection required by the *Life Safety Code*.®

Standard

EC.2.5.1 Management activities temporarily compensate for life-safety deficiencies and construction hazards.

Intent of EC.2.5.1

Each organization must develop a policy for interim life safety measures (ILSM*) that includes written criteria to evaluate various deficiencies and construction hazards for determining when and to what extent one or more of the following measures are applicable:

a. Ensuring free and unobstructed exits. Staff get additional training when alternative exits are designated. Buildings or areas under construction must maintain escape routes for construction workers at all times, and the means of exiting construction areas are inspected daily.
b. Ensuring free and unobstructed access to emergency services and for fire, police, and other emergency forces.
c. Ensuring that fire alarm, detection, and suppression systems are in good working order. A temporary but equivalent system must be provided when any fire system is impaired. Temporary systems must be inspected and tested monthly.

    Note: *The NFPA 101,* Life Safety Code®, *requires that the municipal fire department is notified (or applicable emergency forces group) and a fire watch is provided whenever an approved fire alarm or automatic sprinkler system is out of service for more than 4 hours in a 24-hour period in an occupied building.*
d. Ensuring that temporary construction partitions are smoke-tight and built of noncombustible or limited combustible materials that will not contribute to the development or spread of fire.
e. Providing additional fire-fighting equipment and training staff in its use.
f. Prohibiting smoking (according to EC.2.8.3) throughout the organization's buildings and in and near construction areas.
g. Developing and enforcing storage, housekeeping, and debris-removal practices that reduce the building's flammable and combustible fire load to the lowest feasible level.
h. Conducting a minimum of two fire drills per shift per quarter.
i. Increasing hazard surveillance of buildings, grounds, and equipment, with special attention to excavations, construction areas, construction storage, and field offices.
j. Training staff to compensate for impaired structural or compartmentalization features of fire safety.
k. Conducting organizationwide safety education programs to promote awareness of *LSC®* deficiencies, construction hazards, and ILSM.

---

* **interim life safety measures (ILSM)** A series of 11 administrative actions required to temporarily compensate for significant hazards posed by existing life-safety deficiencies or construction activities. ILSM apply to appropriate staff (including construction workers), must be implemented upon project development, and must be continuously enforced through project completion. Each ILSM action must be documented through written policies and procedures. Frequencies for inspection, testing, training, and monitoring and evaluation must be established by the organization.

Standard

EC.2.5.2 The environment is designed and maintained to comply with the *Life Safety Code.*®*

This standard applies to all buildings (owned, operated or leased by the organization) in which individuals served are housed or treated, except for buildings:

- *housing three or less individuals served (see note to EC.2.5a); and*
- *classified as a business occupancy by the* Life Safety Code.®

Intent of EC.2.5.2

Each building in which individuals served are housed

- prepares and maintains a current, organizationwide Statement of Conditions™ (SOC™)†;
- complies with the *Life Safety Code*® (*LSC*®), NFPA 101®–1997;

OR

- does not comply with the *LSC*® but proof that all deficiencies have been resolved is shown by one of the following:
  - An equivalency approved by the Joint Commission; or
  - Continued progress in completing an acceptable Plan For Improvement (SOC™–Part 4).

Note: *A copy of the SOC™ appears at the end of this chapter. You may make as many copies of this SOC™ as you wish. However, remember to keep the original blank for future copying purposes.*

Standard

EC.2.6 A management plan addresses medical equipment.‡

Intent of EC.2.6

A plan describes how the organization establishes and maintains a medical equipment management program to promote safe and effective use of medical equipment. The plan provides processes for

a. selecting and acquiring medical equipment;
b. establishing criteria for identifying, evaluating, and taking inventory of equipment to be included in the management program before the equipment is used; these criteria address
   - equipment function,
   - risks associated with use,
   - maintenance requirements, and
   - equipment incident history;
c. minimizing clinical and physical risks of equipment use through inspection, testing, and maintenance;
d. monitoring and acting on equipment hazard notices and recalls;

---

* NFPA 101, *Life Safety Code*® (*LSC*®) is a registered trademark of the National Fire Protection Association, Inc, Quincy, Massachusetts. Effective January 1, 1998, the Joint Commission began referencing the 1997 edition *LSC*® of the National Fire Protection Association. All facilities being surveyed will be evaluated using the 1997 edition of the *LSC*®. Buildings for which plans were approved after January 1, 1998, will be evaluated as "new construction" under the applicable occupancy chapters of the 1997 edition of the *LSC*®.

† **Statement of Conditions™ compliance document** A proactive document that helps an organization to do a critical self-assessment of its current level of compliance and describe how to resolve any *Life Safety Code*® (*LSC*®) deficiencies. The SOC™ was created to be a "living, ongoing" management tool that should be used in a management process that continually identifies, assesses, and resolves *LSC*® deficiencies.

‡ Medical equipment includes equipment used for diagnosis, treatment, and monitoring of individuals served.

e. monitoring and reporting incidents in which a medical device is connected with the death, serious injury, or serious illness of any individual, as required by the Safe Medical Devices Act of 1990;
f. investigating equipment problems, failures, and user errors;
g. an orientation and education program addressing equipment management;
h. ongoing monitoring of performance regarding actual or potential risks related to one or more of the following:
   - Staff knowledge and skills
   - Level of staff participation
   - Monitoring and inspection activities
   - Emergency and incident reporting
   - Inspection, preventive maintenance, and testing of equipment;
i. emergency procedures that address medical equipment disruptions or failures; and
j. evaluating the medical equipment management plan annually.

A historical record is maintained for each instrument or piece of equipment in the organization. Detailed records identifying daily, weekly, or monthly performance testing and function checks are kept for at least three years, and records of major repairs, parts replacement, and annual maintenance are kept for the life of the instrument or equipment.

Standard

EC.2.7 A management plan addresses utility systems.*

Intent of EC.2.7

A plan describes how the organization establishes and maintains a utility systems management program to

a. promote a safe, controlled, comfortable environment;
b. assess and minimize risks of utility failures; and
c. ensure operational reliability of utility systems.

The plan provides processes for

d. establishing criteria for identifying, evaluating, and taking inventory of critical operating components of systems to be included in the utility management program; these criteria address the impact of utility systems on
   - infection control systems,
   - environmental support systems,
   - equipment-support systems, and
   - communication systems;
e. inspecting, testing, and maintaining critical operating components;
f. developing and maintaining current utility system operational plans to help ensure reliability, minimize risks, and reduce failures;
g. mapping the layout of utility systems and labeling controls for a partial or complete emergency shutdown;
h. investigating utility systems management problems, failures, or user errors and reporting incidents and corrective actions;
i. an orientation and education program addressing utility systems management;

---

* **utility systems** Organization systems for surveillance, prevention, and control of infection, environment support, and equipment support. May include electrical distribution, emergency power, vertical and horizontal transport. Heating, ventilating and air conditioning, plumbing, boiler and steam, piped gases, vacuum systems, or communication systems including data exchange systems.

j. ongoing monitoring of performance regarding actual or potential risks related to one or more of the following:
   - Staff knowledge and skills
   - Level of staff participation
   - Monitoring and inspection activities
   - Emergency and incident reporting
   - Inspection, preventive maintenance, and testing of equipment;

k. emergency procedures for utility system disruptions or failures; and

l. evaluating the utility management plan annually.

The organization also

m. provides a reliable emergency power system, when required by occupancy classification, that supplies electricity to the following areas when normal electricity is interrupted:
   - Alarm systems,
   - Exit route illumination (including illumination of exit signs), and
   - Emergency communication systems; and

n. if needed because of item "m," properly installs an emergency power source that is adequately sized, designed, and fueled.

Standard

EC.2.8 *A management plan addresses the physical environment.*

Intent of EC.2.8

In designing the organization's environment, other factors besides those listed in EC.2.1 through EC.2.7 may also apply to the environment. These are addressed in EC.2.8.1 through EC.2.8.3.

Standard

EC.2.8.1 When designing the environment, the organization uses design criteria from the health care community.

Intent of EC.2.8.1

When planning the size, configuration, and equipping of space of renovated, altered, or new construction, the organization uses

- *Guidelines for Design and Construction of Hospitals and Health Care Facilities,* 1996 edition, published by the American Institute of Architects; or
- state rules and regulations; or
- similar standards or guidelines.

When site conditions or specific clinical needs require deviation from the guidelines or standards cited here, the organization identifies, when appropriate, needs for specialized staff training to effectively use the space and equipment provided.

Standard

EC.2.8.2 The organization has enough space and equipment for staff to provide the services offered.

Intent of EC.2.8.2

Care should not be adversely affected by inappropriate or insufficient equipment or inappropriate provisions for equipment, and there should be enough space for staff to provide the services offered. The space-allocation management plan describes how the organization will establish and maintain a program that supplies adequate space. The plan provides processes for

- providing interior and exterior space suitable to the nature of the clinical services offered and the ages and other characteristics of the population served;
- ensuring the safe use, maintenance, and supervision of grounds, equipment (both medical and nonmedical), and special activity areas; and
- performance standards for staff members' space-management knowledge.

Standard

EC.2.8.3 A policy prohibiting smoking is developed.

Intent of EC.2.8.3

Individuals served, visitors, and staff are prohibited from smoking in any of the organization's buildings. These standards are intended to restrict smoking to a minimum and reduce risks of

a. disease;
b. passive smoking from others; and
c. fire.

The organization prohibits smoking (no clinical exceptions allowed) for all organization-based outpatient care services and for all child or adolescent individuals. Visitors and staff within the organization's building(s) may not smoke.

However, there may be clinical reasons to permit some adults served to smoke while in the organization (for example, if sudden withdrawal may interfere with the individual's treatment). The smoking policy provides for such exceptions when they are based on criteria defined by the clinical staff and when they are authorized by a licensed independent practitioner.

Settings that provide longer term care may have a policy that allows individuals to smoke without a licensed independent practitioner's written authorization. In these instances, smoking occurs in designated locations that are environmentally separate from all care areas. Settings that provide longer term care for the following populations are included under this provision:

- chronically mentally ill individuals;
- long term or intermediate care and skilled nursing individuals;
- forensic psychiatry individuals; and
- postacute head trauma (social rehabilitation) individuals.

When the organization allows these populations to smoke,

- smoking may occur within the organization's building(s);
- the organization minimizes the smoke to the extent reasonably possible;
- the organization discourages all such smoking; and
- the organization provides education and options for smoking cessation activities.

These standards do not require that a designated smoking area be a specific distance from care areas. A separate, well-ventilated room (such as a designated smoking lounge for authorized smoking) is an acceptable smoking area.

Standard

EC.2.9 An organizationwide Information Collection and Evaluation System is developed.

Intent of EC.2.9

The Information Collection and Evaluation System (ICES) aggregates information from all major components of the organization's environment. Data are collected about implementation of all management programs described in EC.2.1 through EC.2.8.3. EC.3.2 describes how the ICES is carried out.

Implementation

Standard

EC.3 *The organization provides a safe, accessible, effective, and efficient environment consistent with its mission, services, and law and regulation through training, drills, performance, and maintenance.*

Intent of EC.3

Each organization has an active safety program to the degree required by the risks and hazards encountered in the organization. The program carries out safety practices and prevention measures for staff, individuals served, and visitors.

Standard

EC.3.1 The management plans are carried out.

Intent of EC.3.1

The organization carries out the management plans addressed in EC.2.1 through EC.2.8.3 for

a. safety management,
b. security management,
c. hazardous materials and wastes management,
d. emergency preparedness management,
e. life safety management,
f. medical equipment management,
g. utility systems management, and
h. physical environment (smoking, space, equipment).

Standard

EC.3.1.1 Staff have been oriented to and educated about the environment and have the knowledge and skills to perform their responsibilities under the management plans.*

---

* As described in EC.2.1 through EC.2.9, the organization has management plans for the following factors in the environment: safety, security, hazardous materials and wastes, emergency preparedness, life safety, medical equipment, utility systems, other physical environmental considerations, and a data collection system.

Intent of EC.3.1.1

Each staff member is oriented to appropriate environment of care procedures and practices. Established performance standards measure staff knowledge and skill related to their roles in the safety program; roles in the findings of safety inspections; roles in incident and risk reporting; roles in the notification and recall process; roles in the preventive maintenance process; and correct use of equipment, including required testing and handling of broken or potentially unsafe equipment. Staff can describe or demonstrate

a. safety risks in the organization environment;
b. reporting procedures for incidents involving property damage, occupational illness, and injury to individuals served, staff, or visitors;
c. actions to eliminate, minimize, or report safety risks;
d. organization fire-response needs;
e. organization fire evacuation routes;
f. their specific roles and responsibilities in the fire plan;
g. use and functioning of fire alarm systems when required;
h. their specific roles and responsibilities in preparing for building evacuation;
i. emergency procedures for security incidents involving individuals served, visitors, staff, and property;
j. procedures and precautions for selecting, handling, storing, using, and disposing of hazardous materials and wastes;
k. their roles and responsibilities for emergency preparedness, as applicable; and
l. processes for reporting utility system management problems, failures, and user errors.

Standard

EC.3.1.2 Emergency drills are conducted regularly.

Intent of EC.3.1.2

a. Drills are regularly conducted to test emergency preparedness, as required. The organization defines its role in an emergency preparedness plan, as stated in EC.2.4. The emergency preparedness plan is executed semiannually, either in response to an emergency or in planned drills. Organizations that offer emergency services, or are designated as disaster receiving stations, perform trial runs at least yearly that include volunteer or simulated individuals. Drills are conducted at least four months apart and no more than eight months apart.
b. Quarterly fire drills exercise all primary elements of the fire plan* listed below.† All staff of all shifts, in all areas of buildings that house individuals served or in which individuals served are treated, participate in the drills. The performance of all areas during fire drills is evaluated.

Note: *In lieu of observing all areas of the building, an organization randomly observes different locations within the facility, provided the following are included:*

- *The smoke compartment from which the fire drill was initiated;*
- *Another smoke compartment on the same floor level and immediately next to the fire drill location (if one exists);*

---

* Actual transfer or transport of individuals served and building evacuation are not required. Properly documented actual or false alarms may be used for 50% of required drills for each shift, if all elements of the fire plan were implemented.

† Properly documented actual or false alarms may be used for 50% of required drills for each shift, if all elements of the fire plan were implemented.

- *Another smoke compartment on a different floor level either immediately above or below the fire drill location (if one exists); and*
- *An additional number of smoke compartments, chosen randomly throughout the facility, that is equal to 20% of the total number of smoke compartments involved in the drill (10% may be justified by satisfactory fire drill experience and safety committee approval).*

Fire drills test staff knowledge of

- use and functioning of fire-alarm systems;
- containment of smoke and fire;
- fire extinguishment;
- specific fire-response duties; and
- preparation for building evacuation.

Standard

EC.3.1.3 The operational components of the management plans are maintained, tested, and inspected.

Intent of EC.3.1.3

a. Safety elements of the organization environment are maintained, tested, and inspected. Hazard surveillance surveys are performed in all areas where individuals are served at least every six months and in all other areas at least annually to identify environmental deficiencies, hazards, and unsafe practices.

b. Life safety elements in the organization environment are maintained, tested, and inspected. The organization demonstrates and documents that

1. Fire alarm *initiating devices* are maintained as follows*
   - all supervisory signal devices (except valve tamper switches) are tested at least quarterly,
   - all valve tamper switches and water flow devices are tested at least semiannually, and
   - all duct detectors, electromechanical releasing devices, heat detectors, manual fire alarm boxes, smoke detectors are tested at least annually;
2. Fire alarm Occupant Alarm Notification devices including all audible devices, speakers, and visible devices are tested at least annually; and
3. Fire alarm off premises Emergency Forces Notification transmission equipment is tested at least quarterly;
4. Water based automatic fire extinguishing systems is inspected and tested as follows†:
   - all fire pumps are tested at least weekly under no flow condition,
   - all fire pumps are tested at least annually under flow,
   - all water storage tank high and low water level alarms are tested at least semiannually,
   - all water storage tank low water temperature alarms (during cold weather only) are tested at least monthly,
   - main drain tests are conducted at least annually at all system risers, and
   - all fire department connections are inspected quarterly.

---

* For additional guidance, see NFPA 72-1996 edition (Table 7-3.2).

† For additional guidance, see NFPA 25-1998 edition.

5. Kitchen automatic fire extinguishing systems are inspected for proper operation at least semiannually* (actual discharge of the fire extinguishing system is not required);
6. Carbon dioxide and other gaseous automatic fire extinguishing systems are tested for proper operation at least annually † (actual discharge of the fire extinguishing system is not required);
7. All portable fire extinguishers are‡
   - clearly identified,
   - inspected at least monthly, and,
   - maintained at least annually;
8. All stand pipe
   - occupant hoses are hydrostatically tested five years after installation and at least every three years thereafter§, and
   - systems receive water flow tests at least every five years**;
9. All fire and smoke dampers are operated (with fusible links removed where applicable) to verify they fully close at least every four years††;
10. All automatic smoke detection shutdown devices for air handling equipment are tested at least annually‡‡; and
11. All horizontal and vertical sliding and rolling fire doors are tested for proper operation and full closure at least annually§§.

c. Medical equipment is maintained, tested, and inspected. The organization demonstrates and documents
   1. a current, accurate, unique inventory of all equipment in the medical equipment management program, regardless of ownership;
   2. that each piece of equipment in the program is tested before its initial use and at least annually thereafter; and

   Note: *An equipment-testing time frame longer than 12 months may be justified based on previous experience and approval by an appointed safety person. The specification of an annual testing interval is not intended to be a single standard of testing needs. It is expected that organizations will apply professional judgment in establishing intervals so that risks and hazards are adequately managed.*

   3. that preventive maintenance, inspection, and testing of medical equipment are performed on a schedule based on organization experience and monitoring.

d. Utility systems are maintained, tested, and inspected. The organization maintains, tests, and inspects critical operating components of utility systems and maintains documentation of

---

* For additional guidance, see NFPA 96-1994 edition (section 8-2).

† For additional guidance, see NFPA 12-1993 edition (section 1-10.3) and NFPA 2001-1996 edition (section 4-1).

‡ For additional guidance, see NFPA 10-1994 edition (sections 1-6, 4-3, and 4-4).

§ For additional guidance, see NFPA 1962-1993 edition (section 2-3).

** For additional guidance, see NFPA 25-1998 edition.

†† For additional guidance, see NFPA 90A-1996 edition (section 3-4.7).

‡‡ For additional guidance, see NFPA 90A-1996 edition (section 4-4.1).

§§ For additional guidance, see NFPA 80-1995 edition (section 15-2.4).

1. a current, accurate separate inventory of all utility components in the utility management program;
2. performance and safety testing of each critical component in the program before its initial use and at least annually thereafter;

   Note: *An equipment-testing time frame longer than 12 months may be justified based on previous experience and approval by an appointed safety person. The specification of an annual testing interval is not intended to be a single standard of testing needs. It is expected that organizations will apply professional judgment in establishing intervals so that risks and hazards are adequately managed.*
3. preventive maintenance and inspection of utility systems, according to a schedule based on current organization experience and ongoing monitoring and evaluation;
4. demonstration of the emergency power system's reliability by conducting, if applicable,
   a. monthly testing of each generator for at least 30 minutes under a dynamic load that is equal to or greater than the higher of the following load values (see bar graphs on page 211):
      - ❑ 30% of the nameplate rating of the generator, after applying any applicable rating factors for site conditions, or
      - ❑ 50% of either the calculated or greatest known load on the emergency power supply system (EPSS); and

      Note: *Organizations may choose to test to less than 30% of the emergency generator's nameplate or 50% of the total emergency power supply system (EPSS) load. However, these organizations shall (in addition to performing a monthly test for 30 minutes under operating temperature) revise their existing documented management plan to conform to current NFPA 99 and NFPA 110 testing and maintenance activities. These activities shall include inspection procedures for assessing the evidence of wet stacking.* If diesel-powered generators show evidence of wet stacking, as determined from these inspection procedures, a resistive load bank or additional load test shall be conducted within twelve months (or more frequently if recommended by the generator's manufacturer). The following are the requirements for this test:*
      - ❑ *Duration—until the exhaust is clear of black smoke, but not less than two hours, and*
      - ❑ *Load—greater than or equal to 80% of nameplate.*

   b. monthly testing of all automatic transfer switches; and
5. performance testing of all sterilizers used.

Measurement Systems

Standard

EC.3.2 An organizationwide Information Collection and Evaluation System is used to monitor performance data and known risk factors to identify environment of care safety management issues and make recommendations for resolving them.

---

* As per NFPA 110, section 6-4.2 (1996 edition), wet stacking is a field term indicating the presence of unburned fuel or carbon in the exhaust system. Its presence is readily indicated by the presence of black smoke during engine-run operation.

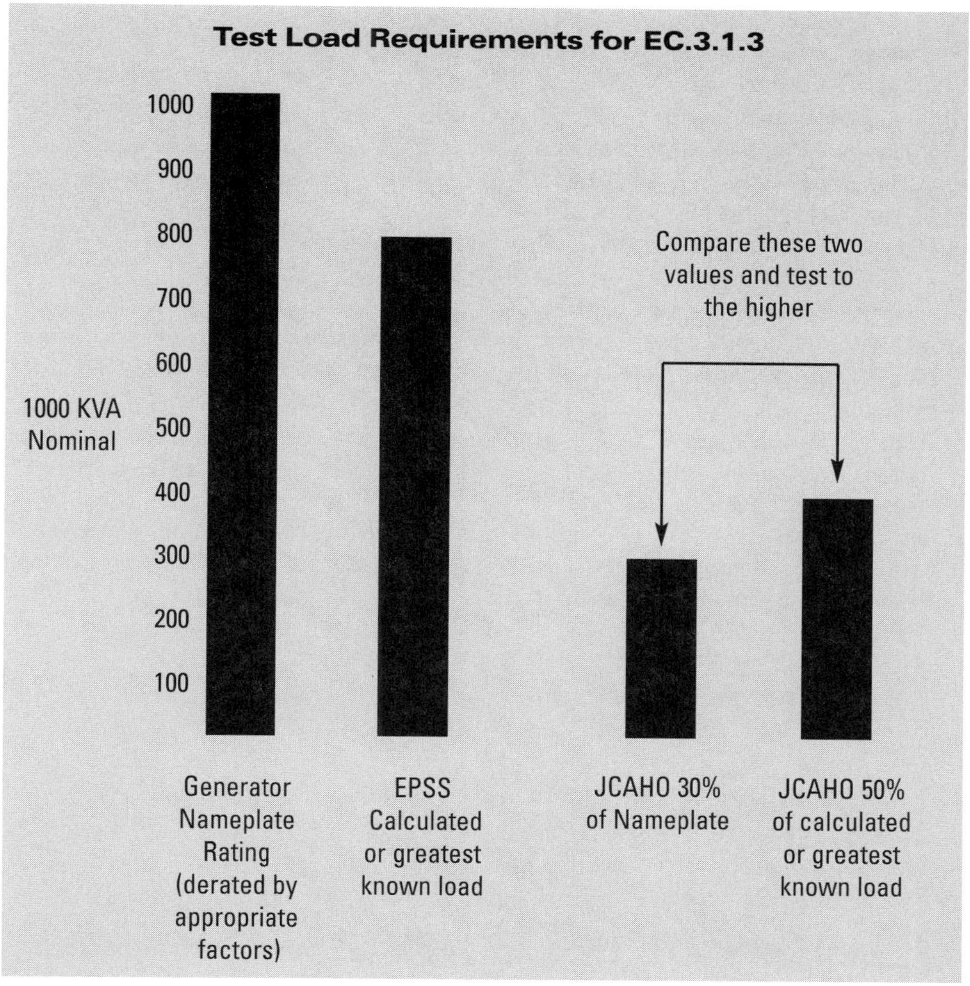

These bar graphs are based on a 1000 KVA generator set with greatest known loads of 800 KVA.

Intent of EC.3.2

a. An individual is appointed to monitor and respond to conditions in the organization's environment.

Note: *When a safety committee exists, it may assume all responsibilities established in EC.2.9 and EC.3.2.*

The assigned individual

1. directs ongoing, organizationwide collection of information about deficiencies and opportunities for improvement in the environment;
2. reviews summaries of deficiencies, problems, failures, and user errors related to management of
   - safety,
   - security,
   - hazardous materials and wastes,
   - emergency preparedness,

- life safety,
- equipment,
- utility systems, and
- physical environment.

3. draws on other sources of information, such as published hazard or recall reports;
4. reports on findings, recommendations, actions taken, and results of measurement to the organization's leadership;
5. regularly participates in hazard surveillance and incident reporting; and
6. participates in developing safety policies and procedures.

b. Safety issues are addressed in a timely manner.
c. Recommendations are developed in a multidisciplinary improvement team (including representatives from clinical, administrative, and support services, when applicable) to resolve safety issues in the organization.
d. Based on the ongoing monitoring of performance in each of the seven management areas, recommendations for one or more performance improvement activities are communicated at least annually to the organization's leaders.
e. Appropriate staff participate in implementing recommendations and monitoring their effectiveness.
f. Safety issues are communicated to the director(s), supervisors, staff, and individuals responsible for performance improvement activities.

Management of Human Resources

Overview

The **goal** of the human resources management function is to create an environment that fosters staff self-development and continued learning to support the organization's mission. Initial assessment of competence consists of reviewing a person's abilities and qualifications* brought to the job. Qualifications and abilities are confirmed as part of the orientation process, and individual competence is later assessed during an individual's performance evaluation.† Staff‡ assess their working environment and provide feedback to the organization's leaders. Improvement of the human resources management function focuses on understanding essential processes and revising those processes based on relevant data.

The essential processes required to carry out this function include

- planning by the organization's leaders that defines the qualifications, competencies, and staffing needed to carry out the organization's mission;
- providing competent staff either through traditional employer-employee arrangements or through negotiation of contractual arrangements with other entities or persons;
- developing and implementing processes designed to ensure that staff competence‡ is assessed, maintained, improved, and demonstrated throughout their association with the organization; and
- providing a work environment that promotes self-development and learning.

---

* **qualifications** The individual's knowledge, competency, training, experience, education, and applicable licensure, registration and/or certification in relation to a specific responsibility and/or position within the organization.

† **evaluation** The review and documentation of an individual's demonstrated ability to achieve the expectations stated in the job description or performance standard.

‡ **staff** Individuals, including employees, volunteers, contractors, or temporary agency personnel who successfully complete a credentialing process and are granted clinical privileges by the organization.

Standards

A list of all standards for this function appears below, presented without footnotes or other explanatory text. If you have any questions about a term used here, please refer to the standard as it appears in the next section of this chapter—Standards and Intent Statements.

HR.1 For their areas of responsibility, leaders define the qualifications and competencies of staff needed to fulfill the organization's mission.

HR.1.1 Staff qualifications are commensurate with anticipated job responsibilities and applicable licensure, law and regulation, registration, and/or certification.

HR.2 The organization provides an adequate number of staff members whose qualifications are consistent with job responsibilities.

HR.3 Competence of all staff members is continuously assessed, maintained, demonstrated, and improved.

HR.3.1 The organization's methods and practices encourage staff self-development and learning.

HR.3.2 An orientation process provides initial training and information.

HR.3.3 Ongoing education and training maintains and improves staff competence.

HR.3.4 The organization continuously collects and aggregates data about patterns and trends in staff competence to identify and respond to staff learning needs.

HR.4 The organization assesses each individual's ability to meet performance expectations, as defined in delineated clinical privileges and/or in job descriptions.

HR.4.1 The organization has a process designed to ensure the competence of licensed independent practitioners.

HR.4.1.1 The process to ensure competence of licensed independent practitioners reviews

HR.4.1.1.1 licensure, certification, or registration;

HR.4.1.1.2 relevant training or experience;

HR.4.1.1.3 current competence; and

HR.4.1.1.4 the ability to perform clinical responsibilities.

HR.4.1.2 Competence and clinical responsibilities are reviewed at least every two years.

HR.4.1.3 Clinical responsibilities for licensed independent practitioners are approved by the governance function.

HR.4.1.4 There is a fair hearing and appeal process for addressing adverse decisions about granting, renewing, or revising of clinical responsibilities for licensed independent practitioners.

HR.4.2 The organization has a process designed to ensure the competence of individuals who provide care under supervision.

HR.4.2.1 Competence of providers who are not independent practitioners is ensured by initial assessment and periodic reassessment.

HR.4.2.2 Providers who are not independent practitioners are supervised on an ongoing basis.

HR.5 The organization establishes policies and practices addressing staff requests to be excused from an aspect of care or service.

HR.6 The competence of those responsible for developing treatment-planning services is determined through review of their education, training, experience, and performance as demonstrated through quality measurement and improvement activities.

HR.6.1 Staff responsible for developing the summary and treatment approach for chemically dependent individuals demonstrate competence in gathering and interpreting information about the dependence.

HR.6.1.1 Staff responsible for developing the summary and treatment approach for chemically dependent individuals demonstrate competence in their knowledge of the natural history of dependence.

HR.6.1.2 Staff responsible for developing the summary and treatment approach for chemically dependent individuals demonstrate competence in their understanding of the biopsychosocial influences and effects of dependencies.

HR.6.1.3 Staff responsible for developing the summary and treatment approach for chemically dependent individuals demonstrate competence in their understanding of the range of treatment needed by such individuals.

HR.6.1.4 Staff responsible for developing the summary and treatment approach for chemically dependent individuals demonstrate competence in their knowledge of available treatment resources and their appropriate use.

HR.7 The process for granting clinical privileges, determining competency, and/or appraising those without clinical privileges for treatment of children or adolescents takes into account the individual's knowledge of growth and development.

HR.7.1 The process for granting clinical privileges, determining competency, and/or appraising those without clinical privileges for treatment of children or adolescents takes into account the individual's understanding of the range of treatment needed by individuals served.

HR.7.2 In organizations where functions of administrative and clinical direction overlap, the individual responsible has appropriate professional qualifications and experience for the population served.

HR.8 Security or correctional staff members may affect individuals' therapeutic goals, so they need to

HR.8.1 know how to respond to unusual clinical events;

HR.8.2 know the organization's channels of clinical, security, and administrative communication; and

HR.8.3 know the distinctions between administrative and clinical seclusion and/or restraint.

HR.9 The staff-development program for staff providing services to individuals with mental retardation and other developmental disabilities includes training in

HR.9.1 proper feeding techniques;

HR.9.2 communication with nonverbal individuals;

HR.9.3 management of aggressive behavior;

HR.9.4 teaching of self-help skills; and

HR.9.5 following of the principle of normalization.

HR.9.6 A qualified mental retardation professional is responsible for coordinating and carrying out services for each individual served.

HR.10 Individuals providing therapeutic foster care services receive ongoing training and supervision to maintain competency.

Standards and Intent Statements

Human Resources Qualifications, Competencies, and Privileges

Standards

HR.1 For their areas of responsibility, leaders define the qualifications and competencies of staff needed to fulfill the organization's mission.

HR.1.1 Staff qualifications are commensurate with anticipated job responsibilities and applicable licensure, law and regulation, registration, and/or certification.

Intent of HR.1 and HR.1.1

An organization's ability to meet the needs of individuals served as defined in its mission often depends on providing qualified, competent staff. Determinations about the organization's staffing needs are based on

- the organization's mission;
- the specific age and disability groups of individuals served;
- case mix of the population and the range and complexity of care required by the population served;
- care and services provided;
- availability of qualified staff in the community;
- availability of appropriate staff within the organization;
- availability of professional nursing care to individuals requiring such services;
- technology used in providing care and services; and
- expectations of the organization, individuals served, families, and customers.

Staff recruitment is based on care and service delivery and organization requirements and is periodically assessed to determine effectiveness. The following elements, as appropriate, are present for each employee or contracted individual:

- Evidence of education and training required by law, regulation and organization policy;
- Evidence of current licensure, certification, and/or registration; and
- Evidence of knowledge and experience for assigned responsibilities.

Standard

HR.2 The organization provides an adequate number of staff members whose qualifications are consistent with job responsibilities.

Intent of HR.2

The organization provides an adequate number of staff members with the experience and training needed to serve and fulfill the program and services part of the organization's mission. Program and service leaders compare projected needs to data and information on current staff numbers and qualifications. This analysis can support, if necessary, proposed modifications for each program or service staff allocation.

The organization establishes staff plans based on

- the needs of individuals served, for example, age and disability considerations;
- organization and program goals and objectives;
- the care and services provided; and
- the need to coordinate care and services.

Generally, programs providing intensive treatment to individuals with severe disabilities will have greater staffing needs. However, no specific staffing formulas, quotas, or models are used for determining compliance; rather, each organization establishes its own staffing plan consistent with its needs.

When appropriately qualified clinical staff are not available or needed on a full-time basis, arrangements are made to get enough staff on an attending, continuing, consultative, or part-time basis.

Standard

HR.3 *Competence of all staff members is continuously assessed, maintained, demonstrated, and improved.*

Intent of HR.3

Staff development needs are addressed on all organizational levels and when planning ongoing staff education activities. Staff are encouraged to participate in appropriate professional associations and continuing educational* activities within or outside the organization.

Competence improvement occurs through formal and informal interaction with peers and colleagues from other organizations and settings. An organization can objectively assess competence in many ways, which means it has a great deal of freedom in constructing its competence-assessment mechanisms. The organization's mechanism, however, must have at least the following two elements functioning to fulfill the intent of HR.3:

1. The competence of staff members is maintained by combining ongoing competence assessment and educational activities; and
2. An objective, measurable competence assessment system is used to evaluate current competence.

For those staff members provided through a contractual arrangement, the organization has on file, for each individual, the job and/or position description and a completed competence assessment and/or appraisal tool. When staff providing care at the organization come from a contracted agency (for example, nurse staff agency, physical therapy agency), the organization defines the job or position and requires the agency to supply evidence that the staff are qualified and competent (such evidence would be the criteria by which the agency assesses competence) or a written statement that contracted staff are currently qualified and competent to perform the duties to be assigned.

Again, how the organization structures these activities is its decision. Whatever mechanism it creates, however, must provide an objective measurement† of each employee's ability to carry out his or her job responsibilities (as defined in a job or position description) in a competent manner, must be defined in organization policies and procedures, and must be followed.

---

* **continuing education** Education beyond initial preparation that is relevant to the type of care delivered in the organization, that provides current knowledge relevant to an individual's field of practice, and that is related to findings from performance improvement activities.

† **measurement** The systematic process of data collection, repeated over time or at a single point in time.

The policies and procedures include a mechanism that determines whether all personnel are medically and emotionally capable of performing assigned tasks (with, if necessary, reasonable accommodation) and free of communicable diseases (consistent with state and federal law*).

Standard

HR.3.1 The organization's methods and practices encourage staff self-development and learning.

Intent of HR.3.1

The performance of any staff member is influenced by how that person's competence interacts with the nature of the work setting. In addition to assessing staff competence, the organization is responsible for creating a work environment that helps staff discover what they need to learn and helps them get new knowledge and skills, as appropriate. Regular feedback from staff helps the organization manage its efforts to create this kind of work environment.

Standard

HR.3.2 An orientation† process provides initial training and information.

Intent of HR.3.2

Each staff member's capability to perform specified duties is assessed by completing an orientation. The orientation familiarizes staff members with their responsibilities and the work place before beginning care and service delivery and other activities. Orientation may also include training in-service unit practices and use of equipment. Volunteers are oriented to care and service delivery, safety, infection control, and other activities for which competent performance is expected.

Standard

HR.3.3 Ongoing education and training maintains and improves staff competence.

Intent of HR.3.3

The organization ensures that each staff member participates in education sessions and training to increase knowledge of specific work-related issues. Staff members' competence is periodically assessed by evaluating the ability to fulfill job responsibilities, especially when new procedures or techniques are introduced and updated technology and equipment are used. Programs have in-service education appropriate to the age and developmental needs of individuals served.

Clinical supervision and consultation are available to clinical practitioners and other staff to maintain and enhance their knowledge, skills, and attitudes in providing care and services.

---

* The Americans with Disabilities Act (ADA) bars certain discrimination based on physical or mental impairments. Toward preventing such discrimination, the act prohibits or mandates various activities. Organizations should examine their hiring and evaluation procedures for activities prohibited or mandates. For example, health care organizations need to determine whether the ADA applies to some or all applicants to their organization. If applicable, the ADA would prohibit an inquiry about the applicant's overall health status. The inquiry must be limited to dealing with the applicant's ability to perform essential job functions, perhaps defined by the privileges or position requirements sought. The Joint Commission has and will absolutely construe these standards to not be inconsistent with the organization's effort to ADA compliance efforts.

† **orientation** A process to provide initial training and information and to assess staff competence related to their job responsibilities and the mission, vision, and values of the organization.

Standard

HR.3.4 The organization continuously collects and aggregates data about patterns and trends in staff competence to identify and respond to staff learning needs.

Intent of HR.3.4

Aggregate data on staff competence patterns and trends are collected from a variety of sources on a continuing basis and analyzed for patterns and trends. The patterns and trends used to identify staff learning needs are acted on by offering in-service education, training, and/or other teaching methods to address identified learning needs. As part of this process, the organization may survey staff to assess competency levels, conduct other similar needs assessment to identify learning needs, and extract data from performance evaluations and performance improvement reports for identifying staff training.

Standard

HR.4 The organization assesses each individual's ability to meet performance expectations, as defined in delineated clinical privileges and/or in job descriptions.

Intent of HR.4

Competence-assessment activities are documented for each staff member, either through the privileging process or an evaluation of performance expectations described in job descriptions. The organization considers special needs and behaviors of specific age or disability groups in defining the qualifications, duties, and responsibilities of staff who have regular clinical contact with the individuals served. Such staff's competency assessments clearly address the age or disability group served and the success with which the staff member can produce the expected results of clinical interventions.

Standard

HR.4.1 The organization has a process designed to ensure the competence of licensed independent practitioners.*

Intent of HR.4.1

Competency-assessment activities are demonstrated for each licensed independent practitioner. Granting privileges or other means to determine the clinical judgement an individual may exercise within the parameters defined by the organization in accordance with licensure law.

The privileging process is not limited to licensed independent practitioners. The standards do not prevent an organization from credentialing and privileging individuals who work under supervision; however, privileging those individuals does not change their status, and they cannot work independently (without direction or supervision) when providing care.

Standards

HR.4.1.1 *The process to ensure competence of licensed independent practitioners reviews*

* **licensed independent practitioner (LIP)** Any individual permitted by law and by the organization to provide care without direction or supervision, within the scope of the individual's licensure or certification and in accordance with individually granted clinical privileges (these individuals may be referred to by other terms such as "independent care provider"). In many behavioral health organizations, LIPs include physicians, psychologists, and social workers.

HR.4.1.1.1 licensure, certification, or registration;

HR.4.1.1.2 relevant training or experience;

HR.4.1.1.3 current competence; and

HR.4.1.1.4 the ability to perform clinical responsibilities.*

Intent of HR.4.1.1 Through HR.4.1.1.4

Professional criteria to determine the clinical judgement that may be exercised by a licensed independent practitioner are specified in rules, regulations, or policies and procedures. Criteria help establish an applicant's background and current competence to provide quality care. Four core criteria are essential to ensuring that all licensed independent practitioners remain qualified and competent:

- Current licensure;
- Relevant training or experience;
- Current competence; and
- Ability to perform clinical responsibilities.

Each credentials file indicates that these criteria are uniformly applied to each individual.

For renewing or revising clinical responsibilities, these criteria could include care and services performed and their outcomes and could be based on pertinent results of performance-improvement activities, as appropriate. Additional criteria may be based on utilization management, meeting and committee attendance, and risk-management data.

The organization may elect to add other reasonable criteria, such as current evidence of adequate professional liability insurance and the applicant's geographic location. Credentials files document uniform application of such criteria.

Appropriate documentation for each of the four core criteria includes the following:

Current licensure. Current licensure is verified by a letter or computer printout from the appropriate state licensing board, or from any state licensing board if the applicant is applying to a federal service. Verification with the licensing board by telephone is also acceptable if this verification is documented. Verification and documentation of current licensure is conducted for all licensed independent practitioners. When clinical privileges are renewed or revised, current licensure is confirmed with the primary source or by viewing the applicant's current license or registration.

Relevant training or experience. During the initial granting of clinical responsibilities, the organization verifies relevant training or experience from the primary source(s), whenever feasible. Verification includes letters from professional schools, internships, residency, or postdoctoral programs. Information from secondary sources is considered supplementary and insufficient by itself to meet this condition. For applicants who have just completed training in an approved residency or postdoctoral program, a letter from the program director is enough.

Current competence. During the initial granting of clinical responsibilities, current competence cannot be determined by licensure, certification, registration, relevant training, or experience alone. Rather, it is verified in writing by individuals personally acquainted with the applicant's professional and clinical performance in other settings. Letters from authoritative sources containing

* See previous ADA footnote.

informed opinions on each applicant's scope and level of performance come directly from the primary source(s). Letters that generally describe the applicant's actual clinical performance, the satisfactory discharge of professional obligations, and ethical performance are acceptable. Ideally, letters also address the following aspects of current competence:

- The populations and outcomes managed by the applicant; and
- The applicant's clinical judgment and technical skills.

When privileges are renewed, current competence is determined by the results of performance-improvement activities and peer recommendations.

Ability to perform clinical responsibilities. The applicant's ability to perform clinical responsibilities must be evaluated, and this evaluation is documented in the individual's credentials file. Documentation may include the applicant's statement that no health problems exist that could affect his or her practice; this statement must be confirmed. Applicants for initial clinical privileges need this statement confirmed by the director of a training program, staff at another organization at which the applicant holds privileges, or by an individual the organization designates. Applicants for renewal or revision of clinical privileges must have this statement confirmed at least by the countersignature of an authorized individual on the applicant's statement.

Organizations verify information about licensure, training, experience, and competence from primary sources (see *Notes* below), whenever possible. An external agency (for example, a local accredited health care organization where the individual is privileged or a credentials verification organization) may be used to collect information from primary sources if the agency furnishes all additional relevant information from the primary source(s). The organization then evaluates the individual's credentials by comparing the information in the application with information provided by the primary source to the external agency. Additional information may be required to fully evaluate each applicant.

It may not always be feasible to get information from the primary source. Occasionally, a primary source, such as an educational institution or a hospital, no longer exists, or the applicant's records might have been lost or destroyed. Applicants may have received education, training, and experience in a foreign country, and for political or other reasons, information on their professional background is not available. When getting information from a primary source is unduly delayed, full clinical privileges are withheld until this information is received. Under these circumstances, the applicant may be given temporary privileges for a limited time in accordance with applicable federal, state, or organization rules, regulations, policies, or procedures. Designated equivalent sources or other reliable secondary sources may be used if a documented attempt to contact the primary source has been made.

Notes:

1. *Designated equivalent sources are selected agencies that have been determined to maintain a specific item(s) of credential information that is identical to the information at the primary source. The designated equivalent sources are:*
   - *The American Medical Association (AMA) Physician Masterfile for verification of a physician's:*
     - *Medical school graduation*
     - *Residency completion*
   - *The American Board of Medical Specialties (ABMS) for verification of a physician's:*
     - *Board certification*
   - *The Education Commission for Foreign Medical Graduates (ECFMG) for verification of a physician's:*
     - *Foreign medical school graduation.*

These designated equivalent sources may be used by the organization or by a credentials verification organization (CVO) used by the organization. There may be other designated equivalent sources for certain applicants, such as for licensure verification of an applicant in the federal service. The organization should communicate with the Joint Commission to determine whether a specific agency qualifies as a designated equivalent source under such special circumstances. The physician profiles from the AMA Physician Masterfile also include other primary source reported information that is similar to primary source verified information provided by a credentials verification organization (CVO). Use of this additional information is subject to the guidelines set forth in Note 2 below.

2. *Any organization that bases its decisions in part on information obtained from a credentials verification organization (CVO) should have confidence in the completeness, accuracy, and timeliness of that information. To achieve this level of confidence in the information, the organization should evaluate the agency providing the information initially and then periodically as appropriate. The principles that guide such an evaluation include:*
   - *The agency makes known to the user what data and information it can provide.*
   - *The agency provides documentation to the user describing how its data collection, information development, and verification process(es) are performed.*
   - *The user is provided sufficient, clear information on database functions that includes any limitations of information available from the agency (e.g., practitioners not included in the database); the time frame for agency responses to requests for information; and a summary overview of quality control processes relating to data integrity, security, transmission accuracy, and technical specifications.*
   - *The user and agency agree upon the format for the transmission of credentials information about an individual from the agency.*
   - *The user can easily discern what information transmitted by the agency is from a primary source and what is not.*
   - *For information transmitted by the agency that can go out of date (e.g., licensure, board certification), the date the information was last updated from the primary source is provided by the agency.*
   - *The agency certifies that the information transmitted to the user accurately presents the information obtained by it.*
   - *The user can discern whether the information transmitted by the agency from a primary source is all the primary source information in the agency's possession pertinent to a given item, or if not, where additional information can be obtained.*
   - *The user can engage the quality control processes of the agency when necessary to resolve concerns about transmission errors, inconsistencies, or other data issues that may be identified from time to time.*

Standard

HR.4.1.2 Competence and clinical responsibilities are reviewed at least every two years.

Intent of HR.4.1.2

The intent of this standard is self-evident.

Standard

HR.4.1.3 Clinical responsibilities for licensed independent practitioners are approved by the governance function.*

Intent of HR.4.1.3

The intent of this standard is self-evident.

Standard

HR.4.1.4 There is a fair hearing and appeal process for addressing adverse decisions about granting, renewing, or revising clinical responsibilities for licensed independent practitioners.

Intent of HR.4.1.4

The organization has a process for providing a fair hearing on adverse decisions about clinical responsibilities for licensed independent practitioners. The organization defines

- how hearing requests are scheduled;
- procedures to be followed during hearings;
- the composition of the hearing committee;
- the agenda for the hearing; and
- how adverse decisions can be appealed.

Standard

HR.4.2 The organization has a process designed to ensure the competence of individuals who provide care under supervision.

Intent of HR.4.2

The competence of individuals providing clinical care under supervision is assessed. The care provided by these individuals is conducted in accordance with documented performance expectations and evaluated through a periodic performance appraisal.

Standard

HR.4.2.1 Competence of providers who are not independent practitioners is ensured by initial assessment and periodic reassessment.

Intent of HR.4.2.1

The organization uses a process to ensure the initial and ongoing competence of individuals who provide care but are not independent practitioners and must be clinically supervised. Determinations of competence are based on education, training, and experience and, when applicable, certification, licensure, or registration.

Standard

HR.4.2.2 Providers who are not independent practitioners are supervised on an ongoing basis.

---

* **governance function** The activity(ies) carried out by the individual(s), group, or agency that has ultimate authority and responsibility for establishing policy, maintaining individual quality care and overseeing organizational management and planning.

Intent of HR.4.2.2

Providers who are not independent practitioners receive case supervision or an appropriate level of clinical supervision for the treatment modalities or services they provide.

A well-defined supervisory process operates with the clinical staff. All appropriate staff (for example, professional social workers, psychologists) have input in determining the supervisory process, which is consistent with the organization's human resource management practices, policies, and procedures. The need for supervision, as well as the scope and depth of that supervision, may be related to age and disability factors.

Managing Staff Requests

Standard

HR.5 The organization establishes policies and practices addressing staff requests to be excused from an aspect of care or service.

Intent of HR.5

The organization respects its staff members' cultural values, ethics, and religious beliefs and the effect these may have on the care and services provided. Organizational processes are designed to ensure consideration of whether conflicting cultural values, ethics, or religious beliefs are enough grounds for granting requests not to participate in care or services. The way such requests are managed is defined in writing and is available for review by all staff. To prevent care and services from suffering if the organization excuses staff from participating in any aspect of care, the organization establishes alternative methods of delivering care and services in these situations.

Policies and procedures specifically

- define which aspects of care and services may conflict with a staff member's values, ethics, or religious beliefs; and
- address how the organization will prevent care and services provided to individuals and their families from being compromised.

Competency Requirements for Special Populations

Chemical Dependency Services

Standard

HR.6 The competence of those responsible for developing treatment planning services is determined through review of their education, training, experience, and performance as demonstrated through quality measurement and improvement activities.

Intent of HR.6

The chemical-dependency program and, if appropriate, the parent organization, evaluate the competence of those responsible for treatment planning. The chemical-dependency program uses objective criteria (training, experience, documented competence) to determine competence to assume specific clinical service responsibilities.

The program continuously monitors and evaluates the clinical performance and competence of those who plan and provide care and services. Performance improvement findings are used by staff and supervisors to determine competence.

Standard

HR.6.1 Staff responsible for developing the summary and treatment approach for chemically dependent individuals demonstrate competence in gathering and interpreting information about the dependence.

Intent of HR.6.1

The individuals responsible for the summary and treatment approach are able to

- gather and assess information about
  - the relationship of each individual's physical status to the dependence,
  - the nature of the emotional compulsion to use alcohol and/or other drugs, and
  - the intensity of the individual's mental preoccupation with using alcohol and/or other drugs;
- interpret information about an individual's use of alcohol and/or other drugs and develop a summary based on an established and recognized system; and
- develop treatment plans based on individuals' problems and needs.

Standard

HR.6.1.1 Staff responsible for developing the summary and treatment approach for chemically dependent individuals demonstrate competence in their knowledge of the natural history of dependence.

Intent of HR.6.1.1

Developing a chemical dependency follows a course that can be recognized by physical and behavioral symptoms. Those responsible for the summary and treatment approach demonstrate an understanding of this natural history of dependence. Such an understanding is critical for distinguishing between alcohol-and other drug-related symptoms and other pre-existing physical problems or pathologic behaviors.

Standard

HR.6.1.2 Staff responsible for developing the summary and treatment approach for chemically dependent individuals demonstrate competence in their understanding of the biopsychosocial influences and effects of dependencies.

Intent of HR.6.1.2

Staff understanding of the biopsychosocial influences and effects of dependencies helps ensure assessment will result in providing care and services that appropriately address the needs of the individuals served.

Standard

HR.6.1.3 Staff responsible for developing the summary and treatment approach for chemically dependent individuals demonstrate competence in their understanding of the range of treatment needed by such individuals.

Intent of HR.6.1.3

Those responsible for developing the treatment approach are able to determine, based on assessment, the most appropriate level and nature of treatment for the dependence. They need to know the acute and chronic nature of the dependence and the ways medical, emotional, behavioral, social, educational, and other interventions are used to treat the individual.

Standard

HR.6.1.4 Staff responsible for developing the summary and treatment approach for chemically dependent individuals demonstrate competence in their knowledge of available treatment resources and their appropriate use.

Intent of HR.6.1.4

Not all individuals, based on their assessed needs, are appropriate for admission to a given chemical-dependency program or service. Many may need additional treatment resources not offered by the program or service. When clinically indicated, staff make these resources available to individuals through referral or other arrangements. When the chemical-dependency program or service is part of another organization, those who develop the summary and treatment approach understand the resources offered by the parent organization.

Child and Adolescent Services

Standards

HR.7 The process for granting clinical privileges, determining competency, and/or appraising those without clinical privileges for treatment of children or adolescents takes into account the individual's knowledge of growth and development.

HR.7.1 The process for granting clinical privileges, determining competency, and/or appraising those without clinical privileges for treatment of children or adolescents takes into account the individual's understanding of the range of treatment needed by individuals served.

Intent of HR.7 and HR.7.1

The organization evaluates staff competence in child or adolescent assessment and treatment. Specialized knowledge and skills are required to understand growth and development in children and adolescents and apply an appropriate range of needed treatment interventions. Objective criteria (training, experience or documented competence) are needed to determine specific clinical responsibilities.

The organization continually monitors the competence of clinical staff providing care and services. Performance improvement findings are available to staff and supervisors who determine care providers' demonstrated competence.

Standard

HR.7.2 In organizations where functions of administrative and clinical direction overlap, the individual responsible has appropriate professional qualifications and experience for the population served.

Intent of HR.7.2

Direction is provided by individuals competent in specialized areas, as required. Training, experience, or documented competence is used to determine necessary clinical and administrative competencies, particularly when clinical and administrative functions overlap for this age-specific population.

Forensic Services

Standards

HR.8 *Security or correctional staff members may affect individuals' therapeutic goals, so they need to*

HR.8.1 know how to respond to unusual clinical events;

HR.8.2 know the organization's channels of clinical, security, and administrative communication; and

HR.8.3 know the distinctions between administrative and clinical seclusion and/or restraint.

Intent of HR.8 Through HR.8.3

The security of a forensic facility usually is maintained by non-clinically trained staff. These security or correctional staff often play central roles in the interactions between individuals served and staff, and therefore can have a therapeutic or antitherapeutic effect. Staff levels in forensic facilities are such that security staff must conduct care activities customarily performed by clinically trained staff. Therefore, in some instances, security needs of individuals may dominate decisions about assigning, classifying, and grouping both facility staff and individuals served within the forensic facility.

Mental Retardation and Developmental Disabilities Services

Standards

HR.9 *The staff-development program for staff providing services to individuals with mental retardation and other developmental disabilities includes training in*

HR.9.1 proper feeding techniques;

HR.9.2 communication with nonverbal individuals;

HR.9.3 management of aggressive behavior;

HR.9.4 teaching of self-help skills; and

HR.9.5 following of the principle of normalization*.

Intent of HR.9 Through HR.9.5

The organization demonstrates a commitment to providing staff who are qualified to address the special needs of individuals served. Staff development includes both initial and ongoing training of direct care staff.

Standard

HR.9.6 A qualified mental retardation professional is responsible for coordinating and carrying out services for each individual served.

Intent of HR.9.6

A mental retardation professional qualified by education, training, and/or experience has the ability to gather and interpret information about a mentally retarded/developmentally disabled individual. The professional understands the individual's needs and the range, intensity, and duration of care, habilitation, or rehabilitation required.

Therapeutic Foster Care Services

Standard

HR.10 Individuals providing therapeutic foster care services receive ongoing training and supervision to maintain competency.

Intent of HR.10

The organization effectively selects individuals providing therapeutic foster care services. These individuals receive ongoing training and supervision to maintain their competency, and their performance and competence is continuously monitored and evaluated.

---

* Normalization is the act or process of making available, to developmentally disabled individuals, patterns and conditions of everyday life that are as similar as possible to those of the mainstream of society, thereby enabling such individuals to enjoy a manner of living that is as close as possible to that considered normal in the community. The basic principle is that what is offered represents the least departure from normal patterns of living that can be effective in meeting the individuals' developmental needs.

Management of Information

Overview

Health care* delivery is a complex endeavor that is highly dependent on information†. Health care organizations rely on information about the science of care, individuals served, the care and services provided, the results of care, and the organization's performance. Because many staff, programs, and services within the organization provide care, access to needed information is critical to providing, coordinating, and integrating appropriate and effective care and services.

The **goal** of the information management function‡ is to collect, manage, and use information to improve individual and organization performance in care and service delivery, governance, management, and support processes. The organization's leaders have overall responsibility for this activity—just as they do for managing the organization's human, material, and financial resources. These standards focus on organizationwide information planning and management processes to meet the organization's internal and external information needs. The key information management processes are

- identifying information needs;
- designing the information management system;
- defining and capturing§ data and information;
- analyzing data and transforming** it into information;
- transmitting†† and reporting data and information; and
- integrating and using information.

These processes are performed in managing

- individual-specific data and information;
- aggregate data and information;
- expert knowledge-based information‡‡; and
- comparative performance data and information.

These standards describe a vision for effective and continuously improving information management in behavioral health care organizations. Achieving this vision involves

- ensuring timely and easy access to complete information throughout the organization;

---

* "Care" includes care, treatment, services, rehabilitation, habilitation, or another program instituted for the individual served.

† **information** An interpreted set(s) of data; organized data that provides a basis for decision making.

‡ **function** A goal-directed, interrelated series of processes such as assessment or care.

§ **capture** Acquisition or recording of data and information.

** **transformation** The process of changing the form of data representation, for example, changing data into information using decision analysis tools.

†† **transmission** The sending of data or information from one location to another location.

‡‡ **knowledge-based information** A collection of stored facts, models, and information that can be used for designing and redesigning processes and for problem solving. In the context of this manual, knowledge-based information is found in the clinical, scientific, and management literature.

- improving data* accuracy;
- balancing requirements of security† and ease of access;
- using aggregate‡ and comparative data to pursue opportunities for improvement;
- redesigning information-related processes to improve efficiency; and
- increasing collaboration and information sharing to enhance individual care.

Management of information is an active, planned effort. Organization leaders assume overall responsibility and specific roles to maintain and improve organizationwide information management. Staff at many levels are educated and trained to effectively use and manage information.

Although efficiency may be improved by computerization and other technologies, the principles of good information management apply to all systems, whether paper-based or electronic.

---

* **data** Uninterpreted material, facts, or clinical observations.

† **data security** Protection of data from intentional or unintentional destruction, modification, or disclosure.

‡ **aggregate** To combine standardized data and information.

Standards

A list of all standards for this function appears below, presented without footnotes or other explanatory text. If you have any questions about a term used here, please refer to the standard as it appears in the next section of this chapter—Standards and Intent Statements.

IM.1 The organization plans and designs information management processes to meet the organization's internal and external information needs.

IM.1.1 Internal and external information management processes are appropriate for the organization's size and complexity.

IM.1.1.1 Direction, staffing, and material resource allocations for information management are based on the scope and complexity of services provided.

IM.1.1.2 Appropriate staff participate in assessing the organization's information needs, selecting appropriate information technology, and integrating and using information systems to manage clinical and organizational information.

IM.2 Information management processes protect the confidentiality, security, and integrity of information.

IM.2.1 The organization determines appropriate levels of security and confidentiality of data and information.

IM.2.2 Data and information can be retrieved quickly and easily without compromising their security and confidentiality.

IM.2.2.1 A written policy allows clinical records to be removed from the organization's jurisdiction and safekeeping only in accordance with law and regulation.

IM.2.2.2 Well-defined processes are used to preserve the confidentiality of data and information deemed sensitive or requiring extraordinary means to protect the privacy of the individuals served.

IM.2.3 The organization effectively safeguards records and information against loss, destruction, tampering, and unauthorized access or use.

IM.3 Uniform data definitions and data-capture methods are used whenever possible.

IM.3.1 Minimum data sets, data definitions, codes, classifications, and terminology are standardized throughout the organization whenever possible.

IM.3.1.1 When available, external systems for standardizing data sets, definitions, codes, classifications, and terminology are considered when developing organization standards.

IM.3.2 The organization collects data in a timely, economical, and efficient manner, with the degree of accuracy, completeness, and discrimination necessary for their intended use.

IM.3.3 The organization assesses data reliability, validity, and accuracy on an ongoing basis and verifies that data bias is minimized.

IM.3.3.1 Clinical records are reviewed at least quarterly for completeness, accuracy, and timely completion of all necessary information.

IM.3.3.1.1 The review of clinical records is performed by the clinical staff, the health information management (clinical record) service, management and administrative services, and, as appropriate, representatives of other programs or services.

IM.3.3.1.2 The review determines that each clinical record, or a representative sample of records, reflects the individual's diagnosis and diagnostic test results when applicable, therapy and services provided, the individual's condition and progress, and condition at discharge.

IM.4 Decision makers and staff who generate, collect, and analyze data and information are educated and trained in the principles of information management.

IM.5 Transmission of data and information is timely and accurate.

IM.5.1 The format and methods for disseminating data and information are standardized, whenever possible.

IM.6 Information management processes provide adequate capabilities for integrating and interpreting data and information.

IM.6.1 The organization determines how long clinical record information is kept, consistent with law, regulation and the requirements of care delivery, legal, research, or educational activities.

IM.7 *The organization defines, captures, analyzes, transforms, transmits, and reports individual-specific data and information on care processes and outcomes.*

IM.7.1 The organization maintains a clinical record for every individual assessed, treated, or served and incorporates information from subsequent contacts with the individual.

IM.7.1.1 Only authorized individuals make entries in clinical records, as specified in organization policies.

IM.7.2 *The clinical record contains enough information to identify the individual, support the diagnosis, justify the treatment, document the course and results, and facilitate continuity of care among health care providers. Each clinical record contains*

IM.7.2.1 the individual's name, address, date of birth, sex, race or ethnic origin, next of kin, education, marital status, employment, and the name and phone number of any legally authorized representative;

IM.7.2.2 the legal status of individuals receiving behavioral health services;

IM.7.2.3 emergency psychiatric and medical care provided to the individual before his or her arrival, if any;

IM.7.2.4 documentation and findings of assessments;

IM.7.2.5 a statement of the conclusions or impressions drawn from the medical history and physical examination, when required;

IM.7.2.6 the diagnosis or diagnostic impression;

IM.7.2.7 the reason(s) for admission or treatment;

IM.7.2.8 the goals and objectives of the individual's care and services;

IM.7.2.9 evidence of known advance directives, when applicable;

IM.7.2.10 evidence of informed consent, when required for procedures and treatments;

IM.7.2.11 diagnostic and therapeutic orders, if any;

IM.7.2.12 all diagnostic and therapeutic procedures, tests, and results;

IM.7.2.13 documentation that individual and family rights are protected;

IM.7.2.14 progress notes made by the clinical staff and other authorized individuals and used as the basis for treatment and habilitation plan development and review;

IM.7.2.15 all reassessments, when necessary;

IM.7.2.16 clinical observations;

IM.7.2.17 the response to care and services provided;

IM.7.2.18 consultation reports;

IM.7.2.19 every medication ordered or prescribed;

IM.7.2.20 every dose of medication administered and any adverse drug reaction;

IM.7.2.21 every medication dispensed or prescribed on discharge;

IM.7.2.22 all relevant diagnoses established during the course of care;

IM.7.2.23 any referrals and communications made to external or internal care providers and to community agencies;

IM.7.2.24 documentation of individual and, as appropriate, family involvement in the treatment program;

IM.7.2.24.1 when appropriate, a separate record is maintained on each family member involved in treatment;

IM.7.2.25 *information on any unusual occurrences, such as*

IM.7.2.25.1 treatment complications,

IM.7.2.25.2 accidents or injuries to the individual,

IM.7.2.25.3 morbidity,

IM.7.2.25.4 the individual's death, and

IM.7.2.25.5 procedures that place the individual at risk or cause unusual pain;

IM.7.2.26 as necessary, documentation of individual, family or guardian consent for admission, treatment, evaluation, continuing care, or research; and

IM.7.2.27 indications for and episodes of special treatment procedures.

IM.7.3 A discharge summary summarizes the reason for treatment or services, the significant findings, the procedures performed, treatment or services provided, the individual's condition on discharge, and any specific instructions given to the individual and/or family, as appropriate.

IM.7.3.1 When individuals are seen for minor problems or interventions (as defined by the clinical staff), a final progress note may be substituted for the discharge summary.

IM.7.3.2 When individuals are transferred to a different level of care within the organization, a transfer summary may be substituted for the discharge summary.

IM.7.4 Documentation for individuals receiving anesthesia includes the following additional information:

IM.7.4.1 the licensed independent practitioner responsible for the individual served records a diagnosis before the procedure;

IM.7.4.2 reports are dictated or written in the clinical record immediately after the procedure and describe the findings, the technical procedures used, the diagnosis, and the name of the primary physician and any assistants;

IM.7.4.2.1 The completed report is authenticated by the physician and filed in the clinical record as soon as possible after the procedure.

IM.7.4.3 Anesthesia documentation includes at least a record of

IM.7.4.3.1 vital signs and level of consciousness;

IM.7.4.3.2 medications administered (including intravenous fluids);

IM.7.4.3.3 any unusual events or complications and how they were managed;

IM.7.4.3.4 identification of those who provided direct care if other than a qualified registered nurse;

IM.7.4.3.5 the individual's discharge from the postanesthesia care area by the responsible licensed independent practitioner or by the use of relevant discharge criteria; and

IM.7.4.3.5.1 Compliance with discharge criteria is fully documented in the clinical record.

IM.7.4.3.6 [*Anesthesia documentation includes at least a record of*] the name of the licensed independent practitioner responsible for discharge.

IM.7.5 Clinical record data and information are managed in a timely manner.

IM.7.5.1 All significant clinical information is entered into the clinical record as soon as possible after it becomes available.

IM.7.5.2 Clinical records are completed within 30 days or less after discharge, as specified in organization policies and procedures.

IM.7.6 Verbal orders of authorized individuals are accepted and transcribed by designated qualified personnel.

IM.7.7 Every clinical record entry is dated, its author identified, and when necessary, authenticated.

IM.7.8 When an individual is admitted to the organization or appears for a prescheduled appointment, the organization uses an information system to routinely assemble all record components. The system also ensures that all record components are assembled in a timely manner, as needed, for individuals seen for unscheduled visits.

IM.7.8.1 The clinical record or computer system alerts authorized users when portions of the record are filed elsewhere.

IM.8 The information management function provides for the definition, capture, analysis, transmission, and reporting of data and information that can be aggregated to support managerial decisions and operations, performance improvement activities, and care delivery.

IM.8.1 Management of data and information that can be aggregated is based on assessed needs. The data and information include at least the following:

IM.8.1.1 When applicable to a pharmacy operated by the organization, pharmacy transactions (as required by applicable law and as necessary to adequately control and account for all drugs) as well as

IM.8.1.1.1 a means of identifying the signatures of all clinicians authorized to prescribe or order medications, and

IM.8.1.1.2 a listing of clinicians' Drug Enforcement Administration numbers, when required;

IM.8.1.2 information about hazards and safety practices used to identify safety management issues to be addressed by the safety committee, including

IM.8.1.2.1 summaries of the deficiencies, problems, failures, and user errors in safety management, life safety management, equipment management, and utilities management, as well as relevant published reports of hazards associated with any of these areas,

IM.8.1.2.2 documented surveys, at least semiannually, of all areas of the facility to identify environmental hazards and unsafe practices, and

IM.8.1.2.3 reports and investigations of all incidents that involve property damage, occupational illness, or injury to the individuals served, personnel or visitors;

IM.8.1.3 Records of any required reporting to proper authorities;

IM.8.1.4 A coding and retrieval system for clinical records by diagnosis and procedure;

IM.8.1.5 A coding and retrieval system for demographic information about individual served;

IM.8.1.6 A coding and retrieval system for financial information;

IM.8.1.7 Measures (indicators) of processes and outcomes for assessing performance;

IM.8.1.8 Summaries of actions taken as the result of organizationwide performance improvement activities, including risk management, utilization management, infection control, and safety management;

IM.8.1.9 The ability to gather accurate, timely information for both operational decision-making and planning purposes; and

IM.8.1.10 Data and information to support research, as desired.

IM.9 The organization effectively uses knowledge-based information in designing, managing, and improving individual care and organizational processes.

IM.9.1 Knowledge-based information systems, resources, and services meet the organization's information needs.

IM.9.2 Design of knowledge-based information services, resources, and systems is based on the care and services provided and the assessed needs of the clinical staff, administrators and managers, other staff, students, individuals, their families, and researchers.

IM.9.2.1 Assessment of the organization's needs for knowledge-based information considers

IM.9.2.1.1 the need for accessibility and timeliness;

IM.9.2.1.2 the need to link with the organization's internal information systems; and

IM.9.2.1.3 the need to link with appropriate external databases and information networks.

IM.9.3 Appropriate systems and structures provide for identification, organization, retrieval, analysis, delivery, and reporting of knowledge-based information and literature to meet identified needs.

IM.9.4 Management of knowledge-based information provides access to clinical and management literature, data in externally produced databases, practice guidelines, and information in multiple formats for individual education.

IM.9.4.1 The organization's knowledge-based information resources are authoritative and up to date.

IM.9.5 All staff has access to current poison-control information.

IM.9.6 A current drug list is readily available to the staff who use it.

IM.10 Comparative performance data and information is collected, analyzed, used, and reported in accordance with national and state guidelines for data-set parity and connectivity.

IM.10.1 External reference databases are used when available.

IM.10.2 The organization contributes to external reference databases when required by law or regulation and appropriate to the organization.

IM.10.3 The security and confidentiality of data and information are maintained when external databases are used.

Standards and Intent Statements

Information Management Planning

Standard

IM.1 The organization plans and designs information management processes to meet the organization's internal and external information needs.

Intent of IM.1

The organization assesses its needs for information management throughout the organization based on its

- mission;
- goals;
- services;
- personnel needs;
- mode(s) of service delivery (for example, partial-hospitalization, outpatient, residential);
- resources; and
- access to affordable technology.

A comprehensive assessment of information management needs considers

- the organization's type, structure, size, and complexity;
- the individuals and groups served by information management processes (for example, governance, managers, clinical staff, individuals served by residential and partial-hospitalization programs, individuals' families, payers and purchasers, regulatory bodies, accrediting bodies);
- information needed for planning purposes;
- information needed for education services and research activities;
- national and state guidelines, laws, and regulations for data-set parity and connectivity in interfacing information systems;
- requirements for internal and external transmission of data and information;
- longitudinal data and information reporting needs;
- internal and external data and information needed to support continuous performance improvement, including measurements of:
    - the expectations and feedback of individuals served and others,
    - processes and outcomes of care, and
    - variations in processes and outcomes;
- information needed to compare performance with internal past performance, with that of other organizations, and with information from the literature;
- the appropriateness of various information technologies;
- the costs of various technologies;
- the need to support customer and supplier relationships;
- analysis of resource use for individuals with particular clinical problems to enhance the cost-effectiveness of care;
- how work flow can be enhanced;
- information needed for clinical and administrative decision making; and

- plans to expand or redesign any services or any long-range plans that are likely to affect the organization's information needs.

Effective processes and systems are developed to manage information within and among programs or services, the clinical staff, the administration and the governing function, and with outside services and agencies.

Standards

IM.1.1 Internal and external information management processes are appropriate for the organization's size and complexity.

IM.1.1.1 Direction, staffing, and material resource allocations for information management are based on the scope and complexity of services provided.

IM.1.1.2 Appropriate staff participate in assessing the organization's information needs, selecting appropriate information technology, and integrating and using information systems to manage clinical and organizational information.

Intent of IM.1.1 Through IM.1.1.2

Behavioral health care organizations vary in size, complexity, governance, structure, and decision needs, so information management systems and processes vary accordingly. The information management processes used are based on an analysis of the entire organization and depend on staff input in a variety of areas and services. The analysis considers what data and information are needed within and among services or programs, the clinical staff, the administration, and the governance structure, as well as information needed to support relationships with outside services, companies, and agencies. Leaders seek input from staff. Appropriate staff ensure that required data and information are available for the individual's care, research, education, and management at every level of the organization.

Standards

IM.2 *Information management processes protect the confidentiality,* security, and integrity† of information.*

IM.2.1 The organization determines appropriate levels of security and confidentiality of data and information.

IM.2.2 Data and information can be retrieved quickly and easily without compromising their security and confidentiality.

IM.2.2.1 A written policy allows clinical records to be removed from the organization's jurisdiction and safekeeping only in accordance with law and regulation.

---

* **confidentiality** **1.** Restriction of access to data and information to individuals who have a need, a reason, and permission for such access. **2.** An individual's right, within the law, to personal and informational privacy, including his or her health care records.

† **data integrity** The accuracy, consistency, and completeness of data.

IM.2.2.2 Well-defined processes are used to preserve the confidentiality of data and information deemed sensitive or requiring extraordinary means to protect the privacy of the individuals served.

IM.2.3 The organization effectively safeguards records and information against loss, destruction, tampering, and unauthorized access or use.

Intent of IM.2 Through IM.2.3

The organization is responsible for maintaining the security and confidentiality of data and information. The conflict between data access and sharing and data confidentiality is addressed. The organization determines the level of security and confidentiality maintained for different categories of information. Access to each category of information is based on need and defined by job title and function. An effective security and confidentiality process defines

- who has access to information;
- the information to which an individual has access;
- the user's obligation to keep information confidential;
- when release of health information or removal of the clinical record is permitted;
- how information is protected against loss, destruction, unauthorized intrusion or use, corruption, and damage; and
- the process followed when confidentiality and security may have been violated.

Standards

IM.3 *Uniform data definitions* and data-capture methods are used whenever possible.*

IM.3.1 Minimum data sets,† data definitions, codes, classifications, and terminology are standardized throughout the organization whenever possible.

IM.3.1.1 When available, external systems for standardizing data sets, definitions, codes, classifications, and terminology are considered when developing organization standards.

IM.3.2 The organization collects data in a timely, economical, and efficient manner, with the degree of accuracy, completeness, and discrimination necessary for their intended use.

IM.3.3 The organization assesses data reliability, validity, and accuracy on an ongoing basis and verifies that data bias‡ is minimized.

Intent of IM.3 Through IM.3.3

Standardization of definitions and terminology facilitates comparison of data within the organization and with other organizations. When available, the organization uses national and state guidelines for data-set uniformity and connectivity.

---

* **data definitions** The identification of the data to be used in analysis.

† **minimum data sets** An agreed-on and accepted set of terms and definitions constituting a core of data; a collection of related data items.

‡ **bias** An influence on results that causes them to routinely depart from the true value.

Uniform application of accepted data definitions, codes, classifications, and terminology supports data pooling and analysis and provides criteria for decision analysis. Quality control systems are used to monitor data content and ensure that data collection is timely and economical. The health care team collecting and reviewing data is responsible for its accuracy and completeness.

Standards

IM.3.3.1 Clinical records are reviewed at least quarterly for completeness, accuracy, and timely completion of all necessary information.

IM.3.3.1.1 The review of clinical records is performed by the clinical staff, the health information management (clinical record) service, management and administrative services, and, as appropriate, representatives of other programs or services.

IM.3.3.1.2 The review determines that each clinical record, or a representative sample of records, reflects the individual's diagnosis and diagnostic test results when applicable, therapy and services provided, the individual's condition and progress, and condition at discharge.

Intent of IM.3.3.1 Through IM.3.3.1.2

As appropriate to the individual served, the review of clinical records addresses the presence, accuracy, timeliness, and authentication of

- identification data;
- clinical assessments;
- medical history, including the chief complaint; details of the present illness; relevant past, social, and family histories (appropriate to the individual's age); an inventory by body system; a report of relevant physical examinations; and a statement of the conclusions or impressions drawn from the medical history and physical examination;
- diagnosis or diagnostic impression;
- a summary integrating the individuals' assessments;
- a statement of the course of action planned for this episode of care or services and of its periodic review, as appropriate;
- diagnostic and therapeutic orders;
- evidence of appropriate informed consent;
- evidence that the rights of the individual and family are protected;
- progress notes by the clinical staff and other authorized staff, including clinical observations and results of therapy;
- consultation reports;
- reports of any diagnostic and therapeutic procedures;
- final diagnosis(es) or diagnostic impression;
- conclusion at the termination of care or services;
- discharge summary; and
- discharge instructions given to the individual and/or family.

A representative sample is one that encompasses all clinicians providing care and services, the organization's full scope of care or services, including the most common populations served, interventions performed, and all high-risk procedures. Samples include clinical records of individuals currently receiving care or services (concurrent review). In addition, clinical records from each physician on the clinical staff are reviewed at least annually.

Standard

IM.4 Decision makers and staff who generate, collect, and analyze data and information are educated and trained in the principles of information management.

Intent of IM.4

Staff are educated and trained to effectively manage, use, and exchange information. All staff who generate, collect, analyze, and use data and information receive such education, which enables them to

- understand issues of security and confidentiality;
- use measurement instruments, statistical tools, and data-analysis methods for transforming data into relevant information;
- collect unbiased data by controlling for confounding or correcting on the basis of acceptable methodologies;
- help interpret data;
- use data and information to support decision making;
- educate individuals served and their families and support their participation in care processes; and
- use indicators to assess and improve systems and processes over time.

Education and training are appropriate to staff members' responsibilities, job descriptions, and data and information needs.

Standards

IM.5 Transmission of data and information is timely and accurate.

IM.5.1 The format and methods for disseminating data and information are standardized, whenever possible.

Intent of IM.5 and IM.5.1

Internally and externally generated data and information are accurately transmitted to users. The integrity of data and information is continuously maintained, and there is adequate communication between data users and suppliers. The timing of transmission is appropriate to the data's intended use.

The format and methods of disseminating internal data and information are tailored to the needs of users and the organization. Dissemination methods and formats allow easy retrieval. Data and information exchange formats are standardized whenever possible to facilitate interpretation.

Standards

IM.6 Information management processes provide adequate capabilities for integrating and interpreting data and information.

IM.6.1 The organization determines how long clinical record information is kept, consistent with law, regulation and the requirements of care delivery, legal, research, or educational activities.

Intent of IM.6 Through IM.6.1

Information management processes make it possible to combine information from various sources and generate reports to support decision making. Specifically, the information management process performs the following six functions:

- Coordinates collection of information;
- Makes information from one system available to another (for example, between clinical and organizational systems);
- Organizes data;
- Analyzes data;
- Interprets and clarifies data; and
- Generates and provides access to longitudinal data.

In addition, the information management process provides the capability to link

- clinical and nonclinical data over time and among all care settings, particularly linking information management processes related to care and organizational functions;
- internal and external information sources;
- individual care data and external databases and bodies of expert health-related, administrative, and research knowledge as well as information from clinical literature; and
- organizational data and management literature.

Clinical Data and Information

Standards

IM.7 *The organization defines, captures, analyzes, transforms, transmits, and reports individual-specific data and information on care processes and outcomes.*

IM.7.1 The organization maintains a clinical record for every individual assessed, treated, or served and incorporates information from subsequent contacts with the individual.

IM.7.1.1 Only authorized individuals make entries in clinical records, as specified in organization policies.

IM.7.2 The clinical record contains enough information to identify the individual, support the diagnosis, justify the treatment, document the course and results, and facilitate continuity of care among health care providers. Each clinical record contains

IM.7.2.1 the individual's name, address, date of birth, sex, race or ethnic origin, next of kin, education, marital status, employment, and the name and phone number of any legally authorized representative;

IM.7.2.2 the legal status of individuals receiving behavioral health services;

IM.7.2.3 emergency psychiatric and medical care provided to the individual before his or her arrival, if any;

IM.7.2.4 documentation and findings of assessments;

IM.7.2.5 a statement of the conclusions or impressions drawn from the medical history and physical examination, when required;

IM.7.2.6 the diagnosis or diagnostic impression;

IM.7.2.7 the reason(s) for admission or treatment;

IM.7.2.8 the goals and objectives of the individual's care and services;

IM.7.2.9 evidence of known advance directives, when applicable;

IM.7.2.10 evidence of informed consent, when required for procedures and treatments;

IM.7.2.11 diagnostic and therapeutic orders, if any;

IM.7.2.12 all diagnostic and therapeutic procedures, tests, and results;

IM.7.2.13 documentation that individual and family* rights are protected;

IM.7.2.14 progress notes made by the clinical staff and other authorized individuals and used as the basis for treatment and habilitation plan development and review;

IM.7.2.15 all reassessments, when necessary;

IM.7.2.16 clinical observations;

IM.7.2.17 the response to care and services provided;

IM.7.2.18 consultation reports;

IM.7.2.19 every medication ordered or prescribed;

IM.7.2.20 every dose of medication administered and any adverse drug reaction;

IM.7.2.21 every medication dispensed or prescribed on discharge;

IM.7.2.22 all relevant diagnoses established during the course of care;

IM.7.2.23 any referrals and communications made to external or internal care providers and to community agencies;

---

* **family** The person(s) who plays a significant role in the member's life, which may include an individual(s) not legally related to the member. This person(s) is often referred to as a surrogate decision maker, if authorized to make care decisions for a member who loses decision-making capacity.

IM.7.2.24 documentation of individual and, as appropriate, family involvement in the treatment program;

IM.7.2.24.1 when appropriate, a separate record is maintained on each family member involved in treatment;

IM.7.2.25 information on any unusual occurrences, such as

IM.7.2.25.1 treatment complications,

IM.7.2.25.2 accidents or injuries to the individual,

IM.7.2.25.3 morbidity,

IM.7.2.25.4 the individual's death, and

IM.7.2.25.5 procedures that place the individual at risk or cause unusual pain;

IM.7.2.26 as necessary, documentation of individual, family or guardian consent for admission, treatment, evaluation, continuing care, or research; and

IM.7.2.27 indications for and episodes of special treatment procedures.

Intent of IM.7 Through IM.7.2.27

The information management system can recall historical data about specific individuals as well as access data about current encounters. Information management processes enable using individual-specific data and information to

- facilitate care delivery;
- serve as a financial and legal record;
- aid in clinical research;
- support decision making; and
- guide professional and organizational performance improvement.

Individual-specific data and information is produced and used by a diverse group, including administrative staff, support services, and direct care providers. To facilitate consistency and continuity in care delivery, very specific data and information are required, as outlined in the standards. Recording and using individual-specific information is timely, accurate, secure, and confidential.

For individuals receiving partial-hospitalization or outpatient care or services for continuing care, defined as three or more visits, the clinical record includes a list of significant diagnoses, conditions, procedures, drug allergies, and medications. The record's format offers easy access to this information, which is stored in the same location in all records to help care and service providers find it quickly and easily before seeing the individual.

The summary list is current and updated as necessary and contains

- significant known diagnoses and conditions;
- significant known past treatment procedures;
- known adverse and allergic drug reactions; and
- currently and recently used medications.

"Known" refers to information gathered as part of the individual's assessment and treatment. If an individual is seen in more than one service in the organization (each of which maintains a separate clinical record), the summary list in each record indicates that there is information in another record.

Standards

IM.7.3 A discharge summary summarizes the reason for treatment or services, the significant findings, the procedures performed, treatment or services provided, the individual's condition on discharge, and any specific instructions given to the individual and/or family, as appropriate.

IM.7.3.1 When individuals are seen for minor problems or interventions (as defined by the clinical staff), a final progress note may be substituted for the discharge summary.

IM.7.3.2 When individuals are transferred to a different level of care within the organization, a transfer summary may be substituted for the discharge summary.

Intent of IM.7.3 Through IM.7.3.2

To concisely provide important information to other users of the clinical record, a discharge summary is included in the record at discharge.

When an individual is transferred from one level of care to another (for example, from residential to partial-hospitalization) within the same organization, and the caregivers change, a transfer summary may be substituted for the discharge summary. When the caregivers are the same, a progress note may be enough.

Standards

IM.7.4 *Documentation for individuals receiving anesthesia includes the following additional information:*

IM.7.4.1 the licensed independent practitioner* responsible for the individual served records a diagnosis before the procedure;

IM.7.4.2 reports are dictated or written in the clinical record immediately after the procedure and describe the findings, the technical procedures used, the diagnosis, and the name of the primary physician and any assistants;

IM.7.4.2.1 The completed report is authenticated by the physician and filed in the clinical record as soon as possible after the procedure.

IM.7.4.3 *Anesthesia documentation includes at least a record of*

IM.7.4.3.1 vital signs and level of consciousness;

---

* **licensed independent practitioner (LIP)** Any individual permitted by law and by the organization to provide care services without direction or supervision, within the scope of the individual's licensure or certification and in accordance with individually granted clinical privileges (these individuals may be referred to by other terms such as "independent care provider"). In many behavioral health organizations, LIPs include physicians, psychologists, and social workers.

IM.7.4.3.2 medications administered (including intravenous fluids);

IM.7.4.3.3 any unusual events or complications and how they were managed;

IM.7.4.3.4 identification of those who provided direct care if other than a qualified registered nurse;

IM.7.4.3.5 the individual's discharge from the postanesthesia care area by the responsible licensed independent practitioner or by the use of relevant discharge criteria; and

IM.7.4.3.5.1 Compliance with discharge criteria is fully documented in the clinical record.

IM.7.4.3.6 [*Anesthesia documentation includes at least a record of*] the name of the licensed independent practitioner responsible for discharge.

Intent of IM.7.4 Through IM.7.4.3.6

In addition to the specific information* required in all clinical records, all aspects and events of an individual's anesthesia care are recorded. The record includes the diagnosis, a complete description of the procedure and the findings, the identity of all clinicians involved in the process, evidence of the individual's readiness for discharge from the postanesthesia care area, and documentation of the discharge.

Standards

IM.7.5 *Clinical record data and information are managed in a timely manner.*

IM.7.5.1 All significant clinical information is entered into the clinical record as soon as possible after it becomes available.

IM.7.5.2 Clinical records are completed within 30 days or less after discharge, as specified in organization policies and procedures.

Intent of IM.7.5 Through IM.7.5.2

The clinical record's value in individual care depends on timely completion of all required entries. All significant clinical information about an individual is incorporated in the clinical record within a clinically appropriate time frame, either manually or by computerized entry. The clinical record is complete when

- it contains the diagnosis or diagnostic impression, test results, therapy, and the individual's condition and progress;
- its contents, including any required discharge summary or final progress notes, are assembled and authenticated; and
- all diagnoses and complications are recorded without the use of symbols or abbreviations.

Standard

IM.7.6 Verbal orders of authorized individuals are accepted and transcribed by designated qualified personnel.

---

* See IM.7 through IM.7.3.2.

Intent of IM.7.6

Processes for receiving, transcribing, and authenticating verbal orders are established to protect the quality of care to the individual served. Qualified personnel are identified and authorized to receive and record verbal orders. Each verbal order is dated and is identified by the names of the individuals who gave it and received it. The record indicates who implemented it.

When required by state or federal law and regulation, verbal orders are authenticated within the specified time frame.

Standard

IM.7.7 Every clinical record entry is dated, its author identified, and, when necessary, authenticated.

Intent of IM.7.7

The organization has a way of

- assuring that only authorized individuals make entries into clinical records;
- identifying the date and author of every entry in the clinical record; and
- enabling the author to authenticate an entry to verify that it is complete, accurate, and final.

The author authenticates those entries required by organization policy. The organization ensures that, at a minimum, entries of histories and physical examinations, evaluations and assessments, progress notes, medication orders, and discharge summaries are authenticated. Other entries are authenticated as specified by organization policy or as required by state or federal law and regulation.

Organizations establish policies and mechanisms to assure that only an author can authenticate his or her own entry. Indications of authentication can include written signatures, or initials, rubber-stamps, and computer "signatures" (or sequence of keys).

Standards

IM.7.8 When an individual is admitted to the organization or appears for a prescheduled appointment, the organization uses an information system to routinely assemble all record components. The system also ensures that all record components are assembled in a timely manner, as needed, for individuals seen for unscheduled visits.

IM.7.8.1 The clinical record or computer system alerts authorized users when portions of the record are filed elsewhere.

Intent of IM.7.8 and IM.7.8.1

To promote continuity of care over time and among providers, clinicians have ready access to information about all previous care given to an individual anywhere in the organization. This information is provided in a timely manner by hard copy or screen display. This information is available when individuals

- are admitted to the partial-hospitalization program;
- are seen for a prescheduled outpatient visit; or
- appear for an unscheduled outpatient visit or emergency mental health visit.

A clinical record system is one effective way to combine records of care generated by different services, disciplines, or subdivisions of the organization. Another approach is to insert significant material, such as the discharge summary, progress notes, and clinical reports, from the inpatient record into the partial-hospitalization and residential care records, or a computer-based record system can assemble information about the individual from multiple databases in the organization.

Aggregate Data and Information

Standards

IM.8 The information management function provides for the definition, capture, analysis, transmission, and reporting of data and information that can be aggregated to support managerial decisions and operations, performance improvement activities, and care delivery.

IM.8.1 *Management of data and information that can be aggregated is based on assessed needs. The data and information include at least the following:*

IM.8.1.1 When applicable to a pharmacy operated by the organization, pharmacy transactions (as required by applicable law and as necessary to adequately control and account for all drugs) as well as

IM.8.1.1.1 a means of identifying the signatures of all clinicians authorized to prescribe or order medications, and

IM.8.1.1.2 a listing of clinicians' Drug Enforcement Administration numbers, when required;

IM.8.1.2 *Information about hazards and safety practices used to identify safety management issues to be addressed by the safety committee, including*

IM.8.1.2.1 summaries of the deficiencies, problems, failures, and user errors in safety management, life safety management, equipment management, and utilities management, as well as relevant published reports of hazards associated with any of these areas,

IM.8.1.2.2 documented surveys, at least semiannually, of all areas of the facility to identify environmental hazards and unsafe practices, and

IM.8.1.2.3 reports and investigations of all incidents that involve property damage, occupational illness, or injury to the individuals served, personnel or visitors;

IM.8.1.3 records of any required reporting to proper authorities;

IM.8.1.4 A coding and retrieval system for clinical records by diagnosis and procedure;

IM.8.1.5 A coding and retrieval system for demographic information about individual served;

IM.8.1.6 A coding and retrieval system for financial information;

IM.8.1.7 Measures (indicators) of processes and outcomes for assessing performance;

IM.8.1.8 Summaries of actions taken as the result of organizationwide performance improvement activities, including risk management, utilization management, infection control, and safety management;

IM.8.1.9 The ability to gather accurate, timely information for both operational decision-making and planning purposes; and

IM.8.1.10 Data and information to support research, as desired.

Intent of IM.8 Through IM.8.1.10

Clinical and administrative data can be aggregated and analyzed to

- support decision making;
- track trends over time;
- make comparisons within the organization and with other organizations; and
- improve performance.

Knowledge-Based Information

Standard

IM.9 *The organization effectively uses knowledge-based information in designing, managing, and improving individual care and organizational processes.*

Intent of IM.9

Knowledge-based information provides authoritative, up-to-date print and non-print resources, including

- current periodicals;
- indexes and abstracts in print or electronic format;
- recent editions of texts and other resources; and
- education materials appropriate to the needs of the organization and individuals served.

The organization uses knowledge-based information to support

- clinical and management decision making;
- performance improvement activities;
- continuing education of staff;
- individual and family education; and
- research.

The processes involved in managing knowledge-based information are

- identification and collection;
- organization;
- retrieval;

- analysis;
- delivery; and
- reporting.

Management of knowledge-based information need not be conducted entirely on site. For example, organizations are not required to have a library on site. Services may be shared with other organizations or community resources, as long as needed information is accessible to staff in a timely manner.

Standard

IM.9.1 Knowledge-based information systems, resources, and services meet the organization's information needs.

Intent of IM.9.1

The organization assesses its needs for knowledge-based information and develops a plan for managing clinical and management literature, reference information, and research data. Information management systems provide access to knowledge-based information needed in

- clinical and management decision making;
- performance improvement activities;
- continuing education of staff;
- individual and family education; and
- research.

Standards

IM.9.2 Design of knowledge-based information services, resources, and systems is based on the care and services provided and the assessed needs of the clinical staff, administrators and managers, other staff, students, individuals, their families, and researchers.

IM.9.2.1 *Assessment of the organization's needs for knowledge-based information considers*

IM.9.2.1.1 the need for accessibility and timeliness;

IM.9.2.1.2 the need to link with the organization's internal information systems; and

IM.9.2.1.3 the need to link with appropriate external databases and information networks.

Intent of IM.9.2 Through IM.9.2.1.3

The library and information services enable the organization to

- respond to information requests from the clinical and management staff, other organizational staff, and individuals and their families, as appropriate;
- anticipate information needs and systematically link knowledge-based information with clinical and organizational processes; and
- provide relevant, current, accurate information within acceptable time frames and in formats appropriate to user needs.

Information is accessible in one or more of the following ways:

- Immediately at the work site;

- In a shared central collection within the treatment setting (for example, a professional library); and/or
- From external sources within acceptable time frames (for example, from vendors or other institutions).

The quality of either proactive or responsive information service depends on response time and the information's

- accuracy;
- timeliness;
- relevance to the request;
- format (ease of use); and
- validity.

Standard

IM.9.3 Appropriate systems and structures provide for identification, organization, retrieval, analysis, delivery, and reporting of knowledge-based information and literature to meet identified needs.

Intent of IM.9.3

To facilitate providing knowledge-based information, electronic or paper-based systems and structures allow

- organizing resources to facilitate access;
- identifying and locating needed information;
- retrieving and delivering information;
- sharing knowledge-based information internally and externally; and
- controlling for uniformity, completeness, and compatibility with bibliographic and other records.

Systems for locating and identifying knowledge-based information can include

- automated or paper catalogs;
- psychological abstracts indexed by author, title, journal, and subject;
- online databases and CD-ROM databases; and
- subject indexes such as Index Medicus and Medline.

Mechanisms for delivering, retrieving and sharing information can include

- access to medical and university libraries at the local, regional, national, and international levels;
- interlibrary lending and use of library networks;
- participation in other local, regional, national, or international systems for resource sharing (for example, the British Library, the National Library of Medicine, local consortia); and
- use of clearinghouses and commercial information services.

Controls for knowledge-based information can include

- classification systems (for example, the National Library of Medicine Classification System);
- subject thesauruses (for example, Medical Subject Headings);
- the Marc format for bibliographic description;
- codes for interlibrary lending (for example, the Interlibrary Loan Code of the American Library Association); and
- agreements, regulations, and written policies and procedures for cooperative resource sharing.

Standards

IM.9.4 Management of knowledge-based information provides access to clinical and management literature, data in externally produced databases, practice guidelines, and information in multiple formats for individual education.

IM.9.4.1 The organization's knowledge-based information resources are authoritative and up to date.

Intent of IM.9.4 and IM.9.4.1

Knowledge-based resources are accessible to everyone in the organization who needs them, and they offer authoritative and up-to-date clinical and managerial information.

Authoritative resources may be identified by using reference materials such as *Selected Lists of Books and Journals for Allied Health* and *Selected List of Books and Journals for the Small Medical Library* (referred to as the Brandon-Hill list for Allied Health and the Brandon-Hill list, respectively), which are published on alternate years by the Medical Library Association (MLA) in the *Bulletin of the MLA.* Databases, publishing information, customer recommendations, and reviews can also help your organization select resources.

Clinical and management literature are available in appropriate formats, including paper or electronic journals, books, technical reports, reference materials, and audiovisuals. Materials for use in educating individuals served can include brochures, articles, pamphlets, audiovisual aids, and models.

Standards

IM.9.5 All staff have access to current poison-control information.

IM.9.6 A current drug list is readily available to all staff who use it (refer also to standard TX.3.1).

Intent of IM.9.5 and IM.9.6

Poison-control information and drug lists are important types of knowledge-based information that must be current and readily available. Poison-control information must be readily accessible for emergency reference. A poison-control center hotline is usually the best source of up-to-date information on poison.

Comparative Data and Information

Standards

IM.10 *Comparative performance data and information is collected, analyzed, used, and reported in accordance with national and state guidelines for data-set parity and connectivity.*

IM.10.1 External reference databases* are used when available.

* **database** An organized, comprehensive collection of data elements (variables) and their values.

IM.10.2 The organization contributes to external reference databases when required by law or regulation and appropriate to the organization.

IM.10.3 The security and confidentiality of data and information are maintained when external databases are used.

Intent of IM.10 Through IM.10.3

The organization uses an external reference database and comparative information to identify variations from expected patterns or trends. When required or appropriate, the organization contributes information to external reference databases, such as national or regional registries. Aggregate clinical and knowledge-based data and information are exchanged with other health care organizations if possible.

Surveillance, Prevention, and Control of Infection

Overview

The **goal** of the surveillance, prevention, and control of infection function is to identify and reduce the risks of acquiring and transmitting infections among individuals served, employees, clinical staff, contract service workers, volunteers, students, and visitors. Infection control is a broad process that is applied to all services and settings. It includes activities to prevent or minimize the occurrence and transmission of communicable disease and ensure prompt and appropriate institution of available prophylactic and therapeutic measures when necessary. All activities related to the surveillance*, prevention†, and control‡ of infections acquired in the organization, as well as infections brought into the organization, are coordinated under this function.

---

* **surveillance** The continuing scrutiny of all those aspects of the occurrence and transmission of infections that are pertinent to effective control.

† **prevention** Strategies to reduce the probability of an individual acquiring an infection (for example, hand washing, immunization, educational activities).

‡ **control** Preventing the transmission of identified infections. (A process is a goal-directed interrelated series of actions, mechanisms, or steps.)

Standards

A list of standards for this function appears below, presented without footnotes or other explanatory text. If you have any questions about a term, please refer to the standard as it appears in the next section of this chapter—Standards and Intent Statements.

IC.1 The organization uses a coordinated process to reduce the risks of infections in individuals served and care providers.

IC.2 *Processes to reduce the risks of endemic and epidemic infections in individuals served, care providers, and employees address*

IC.2.1 prevention;

IC.2.2 surveillance;

IC.2.3 identification; and

IC.2.4 control of infection.

IC.3 Infections acquired or brought into the organization are reported to staff and public health authorities, as required.

IC.4 The organization's infection control program is designed to reduce the risks and improve trends or rates of epidemiologically significant infections.

IC.4.1 Management systems support the infection control program and ensure adequate data analysis, assessment, and interpretation of findings.

Standards and Intent Statements

Surveillance, Prevention, and Control of Infection

Infections can be brought into or acquired while in the organization. They are infections that one individual gets from another, whether from another individual served or staff member, and, rarely, from contaminated food, water, or other environmental sources. For example, an individual coming to an outpatient treatment program "catches" strep throat from an infected staff member, or a program staff member unknowingly exposes staff members or other individuals to hepatitis A.

Three things have to be present at the same time for an infection to be "acquired." First, there has to be an infectious agent—a virus, bacterium, or fungus—present in the organization's environment. Second, the individual has to be in a condition that permits him or her to "catch" the infectious agent—known as a susceptible host. Third, there has to be a chain of transmission whereby the infectious agent moves from its reservoir (an infected person or environmental element, such as a contaminated food or water supply) to the susceptible host. Therefore, infection control programs are designed to prevent the infection from occurring either by preventing or breaking that "chain of transmission" or by improving the ability of individuals to fend off infectious agents, such as those known as vaccine-preventable diseases.

Various types of behavioral health care programs—partial-hospitalization, outpatient, and residential treatment programs—serve different populations that have differing risks of acquiring infections. All decisions regarding surveillance, prevention, and control activities made by the leaders of any behavioral health care program or service are based on the population being served and the special risks for infection transmission that exist in that population.

For example, the leaders of a program serving children or adolescents (such as a therapeutic foster care program or a residential treatment facility serving children) might focus on risk reduction through immunization programs and surveillance for hepatitis B, rubella, rubeola, mumps, and other vaccine-preventable diseases. This prevention of "childhood" diseases is one of the targeted risk reduction strategies chosen by the program's leaders.

However, the leaders of another program serving outpatients might decide to focus its infection prevention and control efforts on other "preventable diseases," such as influenza, tuberculosis, and hepatitis B. Examples of such outpatient programs include those that provide individual and group therapy for substance abuse or eating disorders to individuals over several weeks or months. These programs might focus their infection control activities on identifying these or other high-risk infections in the population they serve.

Each outpatient behavioral health care organization's infection control program should have policies, procedures, or "standard practices" that are made known to the individuals served. Such policies might include not letting an infected individual participate in group activities until he or she is determined to no longer be infectious, so as to prevent transmission to the other individuals in the behavioral health care program.

An effective infection surveillance, prevention, and control program is designed by the organization's leaders and carried out by a designated, qualified staff member. The standards and their intents that follow this overview outline the scope of the requirements to provide an effective program. Examples of implementation provided with each of the standards give further insight into how various types of behavioral health care organizations have done so.

Standard

IC.1 The organization uses a coordinated process* to reduce the risks of infections in individuals served and care providers.

Intent of IC.1

The organization has a functioning infection control program based on proven epidemiological methods for surveillance and prevention of adverse outcomes related to infection. The program is appropriate to the organization's demographics— geographical location, types of services and care offered, duration of stay, intensity of contact, volume of encounters with individuals served, populations served, clinical focus, and number of employees. The program addresses issues that are epidemiologically important to the organization, such as:

- communicable infections, such as sexually transmitted diseases, streptococcus and staphylococci;
- child or adolescent infections;
- food safety;
- maintenance of immunization status for individuals served;
- tuberculosis and other communicable diseases, especially vaccine-preventable infections; and
- employee health activities.

The process to reduce the risks of infections also involves a coordinated effort of those having direct contact with the individual served, other organization staff, control of environmental factors, and agencies monitoring and recording infectious diseases. Those efforts include: identifying problems or potential problems; establishing reporting procedures for identified problems; and providing education for control and prevention. As part of the coordinating process, the organization's leaders assign responsibility for the infection control program to a qualified individual to manage the activities of the function. This clinical staff member manages the infection control program on at least a part-time basis.

Standards

IC.2 *Processes to reduce the risks of endemic† and epidemic‡ infections in individuals served, care providers, and employees address*

IC.2.1 prevention;

IC.2.2 surveillance;

IC.2.3 identification§; and

---

* **functioning process** A process that, when analyzed, is found to be actively contributing to an organization's compliance with the intent of a standard.

† **endemic** The habitual presence of an infection within a geographic area; may also refer to the usual prevalence of a given disease within such an area.

‡ **epidemic** An outbreak in a community or region of a group of infections of similar nature, clearly in excess of normal expectancy and derived from a common or propagated source.

§ **identification** A set of definitions and criteria or mechanisms designed to support infection control process. Also includes microbiological, serological, and immunological laboratory support services.

IC.2.4 control of infection.

Intent of IC.2 Through IC.2.4

A comprehensive program to reduce the risks of endemic and epidemic infections addresses all essential areas listed above. These processes are based on current scientific knowledge, accepted practice guidelines, and applicable law and regulation. They are applied to individual care and employee health activities.

Prevention is aimed at reducing incidence of disease or at intervention before pathological changes have begun. Examples of prevention include educational programs (such as basic handwashing and universal precautions), or protection from specific infectious agents in the form of immunizations, hygienic food handling, cleaning and sanitizing procedures. Interventions at the prevention level can be viewed as the cornerstone of a comprehensive infection control program because surveillance and control exist to prevent further pathological changes and their severity.

Surveillance efforts seek to detect disease or pathology as early as possible. Activities at this level can be termed "screening" activities. In the behavioral health care settings, they could be activities

- aimed at early identification of a specific problem, such as a communicable illness in a residential setting.
- provided for formal screening, such as TB screening for new employees and individuals served.
- performed on a day-to-day level, such as direct care workers being able to identify an infectious illness as early as possible. Individuals served often move outside of the organization on a daily basis, interact with a greater population and then return to the organization. A comprehensive infection control program would reflect that staff had been educated to perform these ongoing screenings.

Early identification of an infection limits the negative consequence to the affected individual. In addition, it offers the organization the opportunity to limit the transmission of the infection to others. Monitoring of surveillance data identifies relevant changes and trends within the organization.

Control activities seek to limit pathological changes at the individual and group level. The individual or individuals who have been identified as infected or exposed to the pathologic agent are treated early. It is important to the individual served and the organization in that the severity of the illness can be diminished and the potential spread of the agent can be contained. The control of infection can limit the number of individuals (both individuals served and staff) who might become exposed to communicable disease. Components of the infection control program at this level might include

- activities related to isolation of the affected individual from any interaction that would spread the agent.
- include referral of the affected individuals for professional diagnosis and treatment.
- appropriate procedures for isolation and continued monitoring of the individual and/or the entire outbreak, if more than one person is affected.

Standard

IC.3 Infections acquired or brought into the organization are reported to staff and public health authorities, as required.

Intent of IC.3

The organization has processes in place for internal reporting of infections to the proper clinical and administrative staff, including the person responsible for program management. Reportable infectious diseases are also communicated to the public health authorities, as required.

Standards

IC.4 The organization's infection control program is designed to reduce the risks and improve trends or rates of epidemiologically significant infections.

IC.4.1 Management systems support the infection control program and ensure adequate data analysis, assessment, and interpretation of findings.

Intent of IC.4 and IC.4.1

The organization's infection control program is integrated with the organizationwide performance improvement process. Data about infection risks and trends and rates stimulate ongoing study to improve prevention and control activities and reduce infection rates to the lowest possible levels. The organization's leaders provide for management systems (including staff and data systems) to meet the specific requirements of the organization's infection control program and support achievement of its objectives.

Behavioral Health Promotion

Note: *If the delivery of behavioral health promotion services is not part of the mission of the organization, then the organization would not be expected to deliver the services. The standards will be scored NA.*

Overview

The **goal** of the behavioral health promotion function is to

- determine the presence and prevalence of emotional and behavioral health disorders;
- decrease the incidence of illness and impaired functioning;
- address the effects of such services on behavioral health disorders; and
- reduce social environment and community risk factors.

Behavioral health care encompasses a full range of services over the continuum of care—including acute care, transitional care, and long term care services for individuals, families, and communities. Traditional assessment, care, and services can also be expanded to include health promotion and education efforts, as well as preventive services, targeting factors that may compromise health and well-being. **This chapter applies only to those organizations which have chosen to address as part of their mission the provision of behavioral health promotion services.**

The standards in this chapter address processes and activities related to

- the efficacy of behavioral health promotion services;
- the appropriateness of behavioral health promotion services to community or population needs;
- the effectiveness of behavioral health promotion services; and
- whether behavioral health promotion services respect the preferences and values of the population served.

Standards

A list of all standards for this function appears below, presented without footnotes or other explanatory text. If you have any questions about a term used here, please refer to the standard as it appears in the next section of this chapter—Standards and Intent Statements.

PS.1 The leaders establish the organization's role in the provision of behavioral health promotion services.

PS.2 The organization's behavioral health promotion services are efficacious.

PS.3 The organization's behavioral health promotion services are appropriate to the needs of the community or population served.

Standards and Intent Statements

Behavioral Health Promotion

Standard

PS.1 The leaders establish the organization's role in the provision of behavioral health promotion services.

Intent of PS.1

The leaders of the organization consider the range of behavioral health promotion services appropriate to the organization's mission, community and population served, and develop a plan to deliver those services.

The plan for delivering behavioral health promotion services addresses

- the organization's role in delivering behavioral health promotion services; and
- how the organization fulfills its role in providing those services.

To devise such a plan, the organization evaluates the community served and chooses behavioral health promotion programs appropriate to its operations and to the individuals served.

Standard

PS.2 The organization's behavioral health promotion services are efficacious.

Intent of PS.2

The organization understands the efficacy* of its behavioral health promotion services. This understanding becomes the basis for measurement and assessment that can lead to improvements in these services. The organization is not expected to establish efficacy for behavioral health promotion services. Rather, it is expected to ensure that it provides those preventive services for populations which the services have been demonstrated to be efficacious. A good indicator of an efficacious intervention is scientifically credible research which demonstrates that the intervention promotes the individual's mental health and healthy behavior.

Standard

PS.3 The organization's behavioral health promotion services are appropriate to the needs of the community or population served.

Intent of PS.3

To determine the appropriateness of behavioral health promotion services, the organization assesses the needs of the community or population it serves. The organization may conduct the assessment in collaboration with other organizations in the community, or the assessment may be available through other sources (such as other health care organizations, public health departments, or school systems).

---

* **efficacy** The degree to which the care of the individual has been shown to accomplish the desired or projected outcome(s).

No single best method exists for carrying out a community or population health needs assessment. Data collection methods, availability of data sources, and data quality issues contribute to the complexity of the needs assessment process. Therefore, organizations will use differing approaches and methods, and will be in different stages of obtaining community or population needs assessments.

The behavioral health promotion services needs assessment includes at least

a. a definition of the community or population served;
b. the number of people in the community or population served;
c. the distribution of community or population individuals by age or age group, gender, socioeconomic, ethnic and cultural, and/or level of functioning; and
d. an inventory of health promotion services appropriate to the age, gender, community need, and level-of-functioning distributions of the population or community served.

Whom Do I Call?

The following is a list of information resources at the Joint Commission. You can contact the appropriate person by phone, mail, or fax.

By phone: The Joint Commission's main telephone number is 630/792-5000. If you are telephoning, you can also contact the appropriate department directly for the specific issues listed below. The Joint Commission's business hours are 8:30 AM to 5:00 PM central standard time, Monday through Friday. Customer service representatives are available from 8:00 AM to 5:00 PM central standard time Monday through Friday. The Customer Service telephone number is 630/792-5800.

By mail: Mail materials to the Joint Commission at the following address:
Joint Commission on Accreditation of Healthcare Organizations
One Renaissance Boulevard
Oakbrook Terrace, IL 60181

By fax: The Joint Commission's main fax number is 630/792-5005.

Call the Behavioral Health Care department at 630/792-5788 or 630/792-3003 if you have a question about

- application for survey for behavioral health care organizations;
- scheduling of surveys;
- survey agenda or survey process;
- status of your survey report;
- content of your survey report;
- written progress reports (WPRs);
- focused surveys; and
- surveys of behavioral health care organizations.

Call the Department of Standards at 630/792-5900 if you have a question about

- interpretation of behavioral health care organization standards and
- development of behavioral health care organization standards.

Call Customer Service at 630/792-5800 if you have a question about

- general information about Joint Commission products, services, mission, or history;
- your organization's accreditation status or history;
- obtaining a free Joint Commission Publications or Education catalog;
- orders for Joint Commission publications and registration for education seminars; and
- performance reports.

Call the Pricing Unit at 630/792-5115 if you have a question about

- survey fee information.

Call the Department of Publications at 630/792-5431 if you have a question about

- Joint Commission publications.

Call the Department of Education at 630/792-5398 if you have a question about

- custom education programs.

Call the Department of Communications at 630/792-5631 if you have a question about

- publicizing your accreditation.

Call the ORYX Information Line at 630/792-5085 if you have a question about

- the requirements for the ORYX initiative, the scoring of the requirements, or the effect on the survey process;
- performance measurement systems;
- the technicalities of data submission; or
- ORYX PLUS.

Call the Sentinel Event Hotline at 630/792-3700 if you have a question about

- providing information about a Joint Commission accredited organization;
- the Joint Commission sentinel event policy; and
- self-reporting a sentinel event.

Call the Speakers' Bureau at 630/792-4633 if you have a question about

- arranging for a Joint Commission expert to address your organization's staff on issues of concern.

Information About Other Joint Commission Accreditation Programs

Ambulatory care accreditation	630/792-3002
Health care networks accreditation	630/792-3008
Home care accreditation	630/792-3004
Hospital accreditation	630/792-3007
Laboratory accreditation	630/792-3001
Long term care accreditation	630/792-3005
Long term care pharmacy	630/792-3006

Glossary

abuse Intentional maltreatment of an individual which may cause injury, either physical or psychological. *See also* neglect.

mental abuse Includes humiliation, harassment, and threats of punishment or deprivation.

physical abuse Includes hitting, slapping, pinching, or kicking. Also includes controlling behavior through corporal punishment.

sexual abuse Includes sexual harassment, sexual coercion, and sexual assault.

accreditation A determination by an accrediting body that an eligible health care organization complies with applicable Joint Commission standards. *See also* accreditation decision.

accreditation appeal The process through which an organization that has been preliminarily denied Joint Commission accreditation exercises its right to a hearing by an Appeals Hearing Panel, followed by a review of the Panel's report and recommendation by the Joint Commission's Board of Commissioners.

Accreditation Committee The committee of the Joint Commission's Board of Commissioners responsible for oversight of its accreditation process.

accreditation cycle The three-year term at the conclusion of which accreditation expires unless a full survey is performed.

accreditation decision The conclusion regarding an organization's status after evaluation of the results of a Joint Commission on-site survey; recommendations of the surveyor(s); and any other relevant information, such as documentation of compliance with standards, documentation of plans to correct deficiencies, or evidence of recent improvements. The decision may be accreditation with commendation, accreditation, provisional accreditation, conditional accreditation (with or without type I recommendations), preliminary nonaccreditation, or not accredited.

accreditation with commendation The highest accreditation decision awarded by the Joint Commission to an organization that has demonstrated exemplary performance.

accreditation (with or without type I recommendations) A determination by an accrediting body that an eligible health care organization complies with applicable Joint Commission standards.

provisional accreditation An accreditation decision that results when an organization has demonstrated substantial compliance with the selected structural standards used in the first of two surveys conducted under the Joint Commission's Early Survey Policy, option 1. The second survey is conducted approximately six months after the first to allow the organization sufficient time to demonstrate a track record of performance. Provisional accreditation status continues until the organization completes a full survey.

conditional accreditation An accreditation decision that results when an organization is not in substantial compliance with Joint Commission standards but is believed to be capable of achieving acceptable compliance within a stipulated time period. Evidence of correction must be found through a short-term follow-up survey for the organization to be considered for full accreditation status.

preliminary nonaccreditation An accreditation decision that is assigned to an organization when it is found to be in significant noncompliance with Joint Commission standards or when its accreditation is preliminarily withdrawn by the Joint Commission for other reasons (for example, falsification of documents) prior to the determination of the final accreditation decision (for example, not accredited). Preliminary nonaccreditation is an appealable accreditation decision.

not accredited An accreditation decision that results when an organization has been denied accreditation, when its accreditation is withdrawn by the Joint Commission, or when it withdraws from the accreditation process. This designation also describes any organization or network that has never applied for accreditation.

accreditation decision grid A single-page display of the performance areas that summarizes the standards in each Joint Commission accreditation manual. The grid format allows for the presentation of a numerical summary of aggregated compliance scores for a number of related Joint Commission standards. Each score on the grid reflects an organization's assigned level of compliance for standards relating to a key performance area. *See also* summary grid score.

accreditation decision rules Rules based on grid element scores and specific standards compliance issues that determine the accreditation decision, as well as the scope (which and how many elements require monitoring) and type (focused surveys or written progress reports) of follow-up monitoring required for compliance deficiencies.

accreditation duration The three-year time period during which an organization, found to be in compliance with Joint Commission standards, is awarded accreditation.

accreditation history An account of past Joint Commission accreditation decisions for an organization. The Joint Commission may publicly disclose the accreditation history on request.

accreditation manuals The ten Joint Commission books delineating current standards for specified types of health care organizations, networks, or services. The books are designed for use in organization or network self-assessment. The ten manuals are *Accreditation Manual for Preferred Provider Organizations; Comprehensive Accreditation Manual for Ambulatory Care; Comprehensive Accreditation Manual for Behavioral Health Care; Comprehensive Accreditation Manual for Health Care Networks; Comprehensive Accreditation Manual for Home Care; Comprehensive Accreditation Manual for Hospitals: The Official Handbook; Comprehensive Accreditation Manual for Long Term Care; Comprehensive Accreditation Manual for Long Term Care Pharmacies; Comprehensive Accreditation Manual for Managed Behavioral Health Care;* and *Comprehensive Accreditation Manual for Pathology and Clinical Laboratory Services.*

accreditation survey An evaluation of an organization to assess its level of compliance with applicable Joint Commission standards and to make determinations regarding its accreditation status. The survey includes evaluation of documentation of compliance provided by organization staff; verbal information concerning the implementation of standards or examples of their implementation that will enable a determination of compliance to be made; on-site observations by surveyors; and an opportunity for education and consultation regarding standards compliance and performance improvement.

Accreditation Watch An attribute of an organization's Joint Commission accreditation status. A health care organization is placed on Accreditation Watch when a sentinel event has occurred and a thorough and credible root cause analysis of the sentinel event has not been completed within a specified time frame. Although Accreditation Watch status is not an official accreditation category, it can be publicly disclosed by the Joint Commission.

accreditation with commendation *See* accreditation decision.

activity services Structured activities designed to help an individual develop or maintain creative, physical, and social skills through participation in recreation, art, dance, drama, social, or other activities.

administration (administrative *adj***)** The fiscal and general management of an organization, as distinct from the direct provision of services.

advance directive A document or documentation allowing a person to give directions about future medical care or to designate another person(s) to make medical decisions if the individual loses decision-making capacity. Advance directives may include living wills, durable powers of attorney, do-not-resuscitate (DNRs) orders, right to die, or similar documents expressing the individual's preferences as specified in the Patient Self-Determination Act.

advocate A person who represents the rights and interests of another individual as though they were the person's own, in order to realize the rights to which the individual is entitled, obtain needed services, and remove barriers to meeting the individual's needs.

aggregate To combine standardized data and information.

aggregate survey data Information on key organization performance areas and standards collected from organizations surveyed by the Joint Commission. This is combined to produce a database of information concerning the performance of the organizations during a specified time interval.

aggregation The process by which the scores of individual standards are consolidated into a single grid element score. *See also* grid element score; recommendation, type I.

aggregation rules The specific rules, listed by grid element, used to incorporate all Joint Commission survey findings into 45 grid element scores. The format of the rules is commonly referred to as the algorithm. Aggregation rules are reviewed and approved by the Joint Commission Board of Commissioner's Accreditation Committee. *See also* Accreditation Committee; algorithm; grid element; grid element score.

algorithm A series of steps for determining grid element scores addressing a specific issue. *See also* aggregation rules; grid element score.

anesthesia The administration to an individual, in any setting, for any purpose, by any route (general, spinal, or other), of major regional anesthesia or sedation (with or without analgesia) for which there is a reasonable expectation that, in the manner used, the analgesia or sedation will result in the loss of protective reflexes.

anesthetizing location Any area ordinarily used for the administration of anesthetic agents.

appropriateness The degree to which the care and services provided are relevant to an individual's clinical needs, given the current state of knowledge.

art therapy The use of art and artistic processes specifically selected and administered by a qualified art therapist to restore, maintain, or improve an individual's mental, emotional, or social functioning.

assess To transform data into information by analyzing it.

assessment **1.** For purposes of performance improvement, the systematic collection and review of client-specific data. **2.** For purposes of individual assessment, the process established by an organization for obtaining appropriate and necessary information about each individual seeking entry into a health care setting or service. The information is used to match an individual's need with the appropriate setting, care level, and intervention.

audiological assessment A process to delineate the site and degree of auditory dysfunction using audiological tests such as pure tone air-conduction thresholds, speech reception thresholds, speech discrimination measurements, impedance measurements, and others.

audiologist, qualified An individual who has a master's degree from an audiology program approved by a nationally recognized professional accrediting body; who has completed a supervised clinical fellowship year and passed a national examination in audiology or has the documented equivalent in education, training, or experience; and who meets any current legal requirements for licensure.

audiometric screening A process to screen hearing that may include such tests as pure tone air-conduction thresholds, pure tone air-conduction suprathreshold screenings, impedance measurements, or observations of reactions to auditory stimuli.

authenticate To verify that an entry is complete, accurate, and final.

availability The degree to which appropriate care is available to meet an individual's needs.

behavior management The use of basic learning techniques, such as biofeedback, reinforcement, or aversion therapy, to manage and improve an individual's behavior.

behavioral health A broad array of mental health, chemical dependency, forensic, mental retardation, developmental disabilities, and cognitive rehabilitation services provided in settings such as acute, long term, and ambulatory.

bias An influence on results that causes them to routinely depart from the true value.

bioavailability The relative amount of and rate at which a medication dosage reaches the systemic circulation in a therapeutically active form after administration.

bioequivalence The degree to which two formulations of the same medication have equal bioavailability.

blood component A fraction of separated whole blood, for example, red blood cell, plasma, platelets, and granulocytes.

blood derivative A pooled blood product, such as albumin, gamma globulin, or Rh immune globulin whose use is considered significantly lower in risk than that of blood or blood components.

Board of Commissioners The governing body of the Joint Commission. *See* Joint Commission on Accreditation of Healthcare Organizations.

business occupancy *See* occupancy.

bylaws A governance framework that establishes the roles and responsibilities of a body and its members.

capping A limit on the aggregation of an individual Joint Commission standard score that reduces the severity of its impact on the grid element score. *See also* grid element score.

care The provision of accommodations, comfort, and treatment to an individual, implying responsibility for safety, including care, treatment, services, habilitation, rehabilitation, or other programs instituted by the organization for the individual.

case management A process to manage and coordinate health care resource use in the provision of care and services.

central operations *See* delivery system's central operations.

chemical restraint *See* restraint.

child psychiatrist, qualified A physician who specializes in assessing and treating children or adolescents with psychiatric disorders; who is fully licensed to practice medicine in the state in which he or she practices; and who has successfully completed an approved child psychiatry training program, has been certified in child psychiatry by the American Board of Psychiatry and Neurology, or has the documented equivalent in education, training, and experience.

circuit testing To periodically test, in terms of their conductivity, all alarm initiating and notification appliance wiring circuits that are connected to the main fire alarm system control panel.

CLIA '88 The Clinical Laboratory Improvement Amendments of 1988.

client An individual to whom an organization provides services or that it considers a customer. Clients may include individual, consumer, patient or recipient.

clinical leader A health care professional with overall responsibility to plan, organize, and operate a clinical service or program, for example, the clinical director, discipline chief, unit or service director, clinical psychologist, social worker, psychiatric nurses, and qualified psychiatrists.

clinical privileges Authorization granted by the appropriate authority (for example, a governing body) to a practitioner to provide specific care services in an organization within well-defined limits, based on the following factors, as applicable: license, education, training, experience, competence, health status, and judgment.

clinical record The account, compiled by health care professionals, of an individual's history, present illness, findings on examination, details of care and services, and notes on progress.

clinical record administrator, qualified A registered record administrator who has successfully passed an appropriate examination conducted by the American Health Information Management Association, or who has the documented equivalent in education, training, or experience.

clinical record technician, qualified A record technician who has successfully passed the appropriate accreditation examination conducted by the American Health Information Management Association, or who has the documented equivalent in education, training, or experience.

community The individuals, families, groups, agencies, facilities, or institutions within the geographic area served by a health care organization.

community-acquired infection An infection that the individual being served acquired before hospitalization.

competence or competency A determination of an individual's capability to perform up to defined expectations.

compliance To act in accordance with stated requirements, such as standards. Levels of compliance include noncompliance, minimal compliance, partial compliance, significant compliance, and substantial compliance.

conditional accreditation *See* accreditation decision.

confidentiality **1.** Restriction of access to data and information to individuals who have a need, a reason, and permission for such access. **2.** An individual's right, within the law, to personal and informational privacy, including his or her health care records.

consultation 1. Provision of professional advice or services. 2. For purposes of Joint Commission accreditation, advice that is given to staff members of surveyed organizations relating to compliance with standards that are the subject of the survey.

consultation report 1. A potential component of the clinical record consisting of a written opinion by a consultant that reflects, when appropriate, an examination of the individual and the individual's medical record(s). 2. Information given verbally by a consultant to a care provider that reflects, when appropriate, an examination of the individual. The individual's care provider usually documents those opinions in the clinical record.

continuing care Care provided over an extended time, in various settings, spanning the illness-to-wellness continuum.

continuing education Education beyond initial professional preparation that is relevant to the type of care delivered in an organization, that provides current knowledge relevant to an individual's field of practice or service responsibilities, and that may be related to findings from performance-improvement activities.

continuity The degree to which the care of individuals is coordinated among practitioners, among organizations, and over time.

continuum of care Matching an individual's ongoing needs with the appropriate level and type of medical, psychological, health, or social care or service within an organization or across multiple organizations.

contracted services Services provided through a written agreement with another organization, agency, or individual. The agreement specifies the services or personnel to be provided on behalf of the applicant organization and the fees to provide these services or personnel.

control chart A graphic display of data in the order they occur with statistically determined upper and lower limits of expected common-cause variation. A control chart is used to identify special causes of variation, to monitor a process for maintenance, and to determine if process changes have had the desired effect.

control limit In statistics, an expected limit of common-cause variation, sometimes referred to as either an upper or a lower limit. Variation beyond a control limit is evidence that special causes are affecting a process. Control limits are calculated from process data and are not to be confused with engineering specifications or tolerance limits. Control limits are typically plotted on a control chart.

coordination of care or services The process of coordinating care or services provided by a health care organization, including referral to appropriate community resources and liaison with others (such as the individual's physician, other health care organizations, or community services involved in care or services) to meet the ongoing identified needs of individuals, to ensure implementation of the plan of care, and to avoid unnecessary duplication of services.

creative arts therapist, qualified A person who is registered or certified as an art, dance and movement, music, poetry, drama, or psychodrama therapist by a recognized body, or has the documented equivalent in education, training, or experience, and who meets current legal requirements of licensure, registration, or certification in the state in which he or she provides services.

creative arts therapy Therapy which uses creative arts modalities and creative processes during intentional intervention in a therapeutic, rehabilitative, community, or educational setting to foster communication and expression; promote integration of physical, emotional, and cognitive states; enhance self-awareness; facilitate change; and maintain social well-being. Examples of creative arts therapies include art, dance and movement, music, poetry, drama, and psychodrama therapies.

credentialing The process of obtaining, verifying, and assessing the qualifications of a health care practitioner to provide client care services in or for a health care organization.

credentials Documented evidence of licensure, education, training, experience, or other qualifications.

criteria **1.** Expected level(s) of achievement, or specifications against which performance or quality may be compared. **2.** For purposes of eligibility for a Joint Commission survey, the conditions necessary for health care organizations and networks to be surveyed for accreditation by the Joint Commission.

dance and movement therapy The use of psychotherapeutic movement, facilitated by a dance and movement therapist, to further an individual's emotional, cognitive, social, and physical integration.

data Uninterpreted material, facts, or clinical observations.

data accuracy The extent to which data are free of identifiable errors.

data capture The acquisition or recording of data and information.

data connectivity The ability to link data from different sources or systems.

data definition The identification of the data to be used in analysis.

data integrity The accuracy, consistency, and completeness of data.

data parity The degree to which data are equivalent.

data pattern An identifiable arrangement of data that suggests a systematic design or orderly formation relative to a data set.

data reliability The stability, repeatability, or precision of data.

data security The protection of data from intentional or unintentional destruction, modification, or disclosure.

data set *See* minimum data set.

data transformation The process of changing the form of data representation, for example, changing data into information using decision-analysis tools.

data transmission The sending of data or information from one location to another.

data trend One type of data pattern consisting of the general direction of data measurements.

data validity Verification of correctness; reflects the true situation.

database An organized, comprehensive collection of data elements (variables) and their values.

delineation of clinical privileges The listing of the specific clinical privileges an organization's staff member is permitted to perform in the organization.

denominator The lower portion of a fraction used to calculate a rate, proportion, or ratio. The denominator statement of a clinical indicator is the population (or population experience) at risk in the calculation of a rate. *See also* indicator; numerator; performance measure.

dental services Services, provided by a dentist or a qualified individual under the supervision of a dentist, to improve or maintain the health of an individual's teeth, oral cavity, and associated structures.

dentist An individual who has received the degree of either doctor of dental surgery or doctor of dental medicine and who is licensed to practice dentistry.

department Any structural unit of a health care organization, whether it is called a department, service, unit, or something similar.

detoxification The systematic reduction of the amount of a toxic agent in the body or the elimination of a toxic agent from the body.

diagnosis A scientifically or medically acceptable term given to a complex of symptoms (disturbances of function or sensation of which the individual is aware), signs (disturbances the physician or another individual can detect), and findings (detected by laboratory, x-ray, or other diagnostic procedures, or responses to therapy).

diagnostic testing Laboratory and other invasive, diagnostic, and imaging procedures.

dietetic services The delivery of care pertaining to the provision of optimal nutrition and quality food service for individuals.

dietitian, qualified An individual who is registered by the Commission on Dietetic Registration or the American Dietetic Association, or who has the documented equivalent in education, training, and experience, with evidence of relevant continuing education.

dimensions of performance Nine definable, measurable, and improvable attributes of organization performance related to "doing the right things right" (appropriateness, availability, and efficacy) and "doing things well" (timeliness, effectiveness, continuity, safety, efficiency, and respect and caring).

director A person who directs, controls, supervises, or manages an organization or a component thereof.

disaster A natural or man-made event that significantly disrupts the environment of care, such as damage to the organization's building(s) and grounds due to severe wind storms, tornadoes, hurricanes, or earthquakes. Also, an event that disrupts care and treatment, such as loss of utilities (power, water, telephones) due to floods, riots, accidents, or emergencies within the organization or in the surrounding community.

disaster plan *See* emergency-preparedness plan.

discharge The point at which an individual's active involvement with an organization or program is terminated and the organization or program no longer maintains active responsibility for the care of the individual.

documentation The process of recording information in the individual's clinical record and other source documents.

drama therapy Intentional use of drama and theater processes to achieve the therapeutic goals of symptom relief, emotional and physical integration, and personal growth.

drug Any substance, other than food or devices, that may be used on or administered to persons as an aid in the diagnosis, treatment, or prevention of disease or other abnormal condition. *Synonym:* medication.

drug administration The act of giving a prescribed and prepared dose of an identified drug to an individual.

drug allergies A state of hypersensitivity induced by exposure to a particular drug antigen resulting in harmful immunologic reactions on subsequent drug exposures, such as a penicillin drug allergy.

drug dispensing The issuance of one or more doses of a prescribed and prepared drug by a pharmacist or other authorized staff member to another person responsible for administering it.

drug history A drug history includes, but is not necessarily limited to, the following: drugs used in the past; drugs used recently, especially within the preceding 48 hours; drugs of preference; frequency with which each drug is used; route of administration of each drug; drugs used in combination; dosages used; year of first use of each drug; previous occurrences of overdose, withdrawal, or adverse drug reactions; and history of previous treatment for alcohol or drug abuse.

effectiveness The degree to which care is provided in the correct manner, given the current state of knowledge, to achieve the desired or projected outcome(s) for the individual.

efficacy The degree to which the care of the individual has been shown to accomplish the desired or projected outcome(s).

efficiency The relationship between the outcomes (results of care) and the resources used to deliver care.

electroconvulsive therapy A form of somatic treatment that uses electricity to evoke a convulsive response.

emergency-preparedness plan A component of an organization's environment of care program designed to manage the consequences of natural disasters or other emergencies that disrupt the organization's ability to provide care and treatment. *See also* disaster.

endemic infection *See* infection, endemic infection.

enteral nutrition *See* nutrition, enteral.

entry The process by which an individual is screened and/or assessed by the organization or the practitioner in order to determine the capabilities of the organization or practitioner to provide the care or services required to meet the individual's needs.

epidemic infection *See* infection, epidemic infection.

epidemiologically significant infection *See* infection, epidemiologically significant infection.

equipment maintenance, preventive The planned, scheduled, visual, mechanical, engineering, and functional evaluation of equipment conducted before using new equipment and at specified intervals throughout the equipment's lifetime. The purpose is to maintain equipment performance within manufacturers' guidelines and specifications and to help ensure accurate diagnosis, treatment, or monitoring. It includes measuring performance specifications and evaluating specific safety factors.

equipment maintenance, routine The performance of basic safety checks, that is, the visual, technical, and functional evaluations of equipment, to identify obvious deficiencies before they have a negative impact on an individual. It normally includes inspections of the case, power cord, structural frame, enclosure, wheels, controls, indicators, and so on, as appropriate. It must be performed after equipment is reprocessed and before use by another individual, and also may be performed during use by an individual.

family The person(s) who plays a significant role in the individual's life. This may include a person(s) not legally related to the individual. This person(s) is often referred to as a surrogate decision maker if authorized to make care decisions for an individual should the individual lose decision-making capacity. *See also* guardian; surrogate decision maker.

financial audit An independent review certifying that an organization's financial reports reflect its financial status.

first-generation type I recommendation *See* recommendation, type I.

focused survey A survey conducted during the Joint Commission accreditation cycle to assess the degree to which an organization has improved its level of compliance relating to specific recommendations. The subject matter of the survey is typically an area(s) of identified deficiency in compliance; however, other performance areas may also be assessed by a surveyor(s), even though they may not have been previously identified as deficiencies. *See also* compliance; recommendation.

forensic program or service An identified program or service (for example, jail or prison mental health services, court evaluation centers, outpatient probation, parole services) that provides diagnosis, evaluation, or services mandated by the legal/corrections system.

function A goal-directed, interrelated series of processes, such as continuum of care or management of information.

goal An expected result or condition that takes time to achieve and is specified in a measurable statement offering guidance in establishing intermediate objectives toward reaching the goal.

governing body The individual(s), group, or agency that has ultimate authority and responsibility for establishing policy, maintaining care quality, and providing for organization management and planning; other names for this group include the board, board of trustees, board of governors, board of commissioners, and partners (networks).

grid element A performance area that receives a discrete score on the Joint Commission accreditation decision grid. *See also* grid element score; summary grid score.

grid element score A number representing the aggregated scores of individual standards in a grid element. *See also* summary grid score.

guardian A parent, trustee, conservator, committee, or other individual or agency empowered by law to act on behalf of or be responsible for an individual. *See also* family; surrogate decision maker.

hazardous materials and wastes Materials whose handling, use, and storage are guided or defined by local, state, or federal regulation (for example, the Occupational Safety and Health Administration's Regulations for Bloodborne Pathogens regarding the disposal of blood and blood-soaked items; the Nuclear Regulatory Commission's regulations for the handling and disposal of radioactive waste), hazardous vapors (for example, glutaraldehyde, ethylene oxide, nitrous oxide), and hazardous energy sources (for example, ionizing or nonionizing radiation, lasers, microwave, ultrasound). Though the Joint Commission considers infectious waste as falling into this category of materials, federal regulations do not define infectious or medical waste as hazardous waste.

hazardous materials and waste management process or program A management process or program that includes all materials and waste that require special handling in order to address identified occupational and environmental hazards. Infectious waste and medical waste fall into the special handling category since there are recognized occupational exposure issues that must be dealt with properly. The program is expanded, when appropriate, to residential occupancies.

health care occupancy *See* occupancy.

health care organization A generic term used to describe many types of organizations that provide health care services.

histogram A graphic display, using a bar graph, of the frequency distribution of a variable. Rectangles are drawn so that their bases lie on a linear scale representing different intervals, and their heights are proportional to the frequencies of the values within each of the intervals.

human subject research The use of individuals in the systematic study, observation, or evaluation of factors on preventing, assessing, treating, and understanding an illness. The term applies to all behavioral and medical experimental research that involves human beings as experimental subjects.

important process On the basis of evidence or expert consensus, a process which, when operating well, increases the probability that desired outcomes will occur.

improve To take actions that result in the desired measurable change.

incident report Documentation of an event that varies from established policies and procedures for care or service.

independent practitioner *See* licensed independent practitioner.

indicator A measure used to determine, over time, an organization's performance of functions, processes, and outcomes. *See also* denominator; numerator; performance measure.

individual A person who receives treatment services. The term is synonymous with patient, client, resident, consumer, individual served, and recipient of treatment services.

infection An illness produced by a microorganism or other infectious agent.

endemic infection The habitual presence of an infection within a geographic area; may also refer to the usual prevalence of a given disease within such an area.

epidemic infection An outbreak in a community or region of a group of infections of similar nature, clearly in excess of normal expectancy and derived from a common or propagated source.

epidemiologically significant infection An outbreak in a community or region of a group of similar infections that is statistically in excess of normal expectations.

nosocomial infection An infection acquired by an individual while receiving care or services in the health care organization.

nosocomial infection rate The ratio describing the number of individuals with nosocomial infections divided by the number of individuals at risk of developing nosocomial infections. Rates may be stratified by taking into account certain factors that may predispose a specified group of individuals to an increased risk of acquiring a nosocomial infection (also called rate stratification by infection risk).

infection control program An organizationwide program, including policies and procedures, for the surveillance, prevention, and control of infection.

information Interpreted set(s) of data that can assist in decision making.

inpatient program A program, in a suitably equipped setting not eligible for survey as a hospital program under the *Comprehensive Accreditation Manual for Hospitals: The Official Handbook* (*CAMH*), that provides services to persons who require care that warrants 24-hour treatment or habilitation.

in-service Organized education designed to enhance the skills of staff members or teach them new skills relevant to their responsibilities and disciplines.

intent of standard A scorable, brief explanation of a standard's rationale, meaning, and significance.

interim life safety measures (ILSM) A series of 11 administrative actions required to temporarily compensate for significant hazards posed by existing National Fire Protection Association 101® 1997 *Life Safety Code*® (*LSC*®) deficiencies or construction activities. ILSM apply to appropriate staff (including construction workers), must be implemented upon project development, and must be continuously enforced through project completion. Implementation of ILSM is required in or adjacent to all construction areas and throughout buildings with existing *LSC*® deficiencies. ILSM are intended to provide a level of life safety comparable to that described in Chapters 1 through 7, 31, and the applicable occupancy chapters of the *LSC*®. Each ILSM action must be documented through written policies and procedures. Frequencies for inspection, testing, training, and monitoring and evaluation must be established by the organization. *See also Life Safety Code*®; life safety management program.

invasive procedure A procedure involving puncture or incision of the skin, or insertion of an instrument or foreign material into the body, including, but not limited to, percutaneous aspirations, biopsies, cardiac and vascular catheterizations, endoscopies, angioplasties, and implantations, and excluding venipuncture and intravenous therapy.

involuntary seclusion An individual's separation from other individuals or from the individual's room against his or her will or the will of his or her legal representative.

Joint Commission on Accreditation of Healthcare Organizations An independent, not-for-profit organization dedicated to improving the quality of care in organized health care settings. Founded in 1951, its members are the American College of Physicians, the American College of Surgeons, the American Dental Association, the American Hospital Association, and the American Medical Association. The major functions of the Joint Commission include developing accreditation standards, awarding accreditation decisions, and providing education and consultation to health care organizations.

kit All components of a test packaged together.

knowledge-based information A collection of stored facts, models, and information found in the clinical, scientific, and management literature that can be used for designing and redesigning processes and for problem solving.

laboratory *See* pathology and clinical laboratory services.

leader An individual who sets expectations, develops plans, and implements procedures to assess and improve the quality of the organization's governance, management, clinical, and support functions and processes. Leaders include at least members of the governing body; the chief executive officer and other senior managers; clinical leaders (clinical leaders include health care professionals with overall responsibility to plan, organize, and operate a clinical service or program and may include but are not limited to the clinical director, discipline chief, and unit or service director); and staff members in a leadership position within the organization.

licensed independent practitioner (LIP) Any individual permitted by law and by the organization to provide care and services, without direction or supervision, within the scope of the individual's license and consistent with individually granted clinical privileges (these individuals may be referred to by other terms such as "independent care provider"). In many behavioral health organizations, LIPs include physicians, psychologists, and social workers.

licensed practical nurse (LPN) A nurse who has completed a practical nursing program and is licensed by a state to provide routine client care under the direction of a registered nurse or a physician. Referred to as licensed vocational nurse (LVN) in California and Texas.

licensure A legal right that is granted by a government agency in compliance with a statute governing an occupation (such as medicine or nursing) or the operation of an activity (such as in a hospital).

***Life Safety Code*® (*LSC*)** A set of standards for the construction and operation of buildings, intended to provide a reasonable degree of safety to life during fires; prepared, published, and periodically revised by the National Fire Protection Association and adopted by the Joint Commission to evaluate health care organizations under its life safety management program. *See also* interim life safety measures; life safety management program.

life safety management program An organization's documented management plan describing the processes for protecting, staff members, visitors, and property from fire and the products of combustion (smoke). *See also* interim life safety measures; *Life Safety Code*®.

loss of protective reflexes An inability to handle secretions without aspiration or to maintain a patent airway independently.

managed behavioral health care delivery system An entity that provides for behavioral health care services for a defined population, manages the behavioral health care service benefits for that population, and may also manage the financial risk of providing those benefits. The delivery system includes the central operations, care and service provider organizations, and practitioner offices.

measure To collect quantifiable data about a function or process.

measurement The systematic process of data collection, repeated over time or at a single point in time.

medical equipment Fixed and portable equipment used for the diagnosis, treatment, monitoring, and direct care of individuals.

medical equipment management A component of an organization's management of the environment of care program designed to assess and control the clinical and physical risks of fixed and portable equipment used for the diagnosis, treatment, monitoring, and care of individuals.

medical history A component of the medical record consisting of an account of an individual's history, obtained whenever possible from the individual, and including at least the following information: chief complaint, details of the present illness or care needs, relevant past history, and relevant inventory by body systems.

medical laboratory services Clinical laboratory tests conducted for the patient, either directly by the health care organization or as a contracted service, for the purpose of gathering specific information about the patient's condition. *See* pathology and clinical laboratory services.

medical record The account compiled by physicians and other health care professionals of a variety of client health information, such as assessment findings, treatment details, and progress notes.

medical record practitioner, qualified An individual who is eligible for certification as a registered record administrator or as an accredited record technician by the American Health Information Management Association, or who is a graduate of a school of medical record science accredited jointly by the Committee on Allied Health Education and Accreditation and the American Health Information Management Association; or an individual who has the documented equivalent education, training, or experience.

medication Any substance, other than food or devices, that may be used on or administered to persons as an aid in the diagnosis, treatment, or prevention of disease or other abnormal condition. *Synonym:* drug.

medication-use measurement The measurement, assessment, and improvement of the prescribing or ordering, preparing and dispensing, administering, and monitoring of medications.

mental abuse *See* abuse.

mental retardation professional, qualified A person who has been determined by the organization, based on his or her education, training, or experience, to have the ability to gather and interpret information about a person with mental retardation or developmental disabilities in terms of the individual's needs and an understanding of the range, intensity, and duration of treatment or habilitation needed in the individual's care.

minimum data set An agreed-on and accepted set of terms and definitions constituting a core of data; a collection of related data items.

mission statement A written expression that sets forth the purpose of an organization or one of its components. The generation of a mission statement usually precedes the formation of goals and objectives.

moderate-complexity test A test that meets CLIA '88 requirements based on knowledge required to perform the test; minimal training and limited experience required to perform the test; reagents and materials that are generally stable and reliable and reagents and materials that are prepackaged, premeasured, or require no special handling, precautions, or storage conditions; operational steps that are either automatically executed or are easily controlled; and stable and readily available calibration, quality control, and proficiency testing materials. Test system troubleshooting is automatic or self-correcting, or is clearly described or requires minimal judgment. Equipment maintenance provided by the manufacturer is seldom needed, or can easily be performed. Minimal interpretation and judgment are required to perform preanalytic, analytic, and postanalytic processes and resolution of problems requires limited independent interpretation and judgment.

multidisciplinary team A group of clinical staff members composed of representatives of a range of professions, disciplines, or service areas.

music therapy The use of musical or rhythmic interventions specifically selected by a music therapist to restore, maintain, or improve the social or emotional functioning, mental processing, or physical health of individuals.

neglect An impaired quality of life for an individual resulting from the absence of minimal services or resources to meet basic needs. Neglect includes withholding or inadequately providing food and hydration (without physician, client, or surrogate approval), clothing, medical care, and good hygiene. It may also include placing the individual in unsafe or unsupervised conditions. *See also* abuse.

network An entity which offers comprehensive or specialty services that provides, or provides for, integrated health care services to a defined population of individuals. Networks are characterized by a centralized structure which coordinates and integrates services provided by components and practitioners participating in the network.

normalization The act or process of making available to developmentally disabled individuals patterns and conditions of everyday life similar to those of mainstream society. This allows such individuals to enjoy a manner of living close to that considered normal within their community. The basic principle is that providing the least departure from normal patterns of living can effectively meet the individuals' developmental needs.

nosocomial infection *See* infection, nosocomial infection.

nosocomial infection rate *See* infection, nosocomial.

not accredited *See* accreditation decision.

numerator The upper portion of a fraction used to calculate a rate, proportion, or ratio. The numerator statement of a clinical indicator is the population(s) of the event being measured. For example, number of individuals served in the assertive community outreach program over *x* period of time. *See also* denominator; indicator; performance measure.

nursing The health profession dealing with nursing care and services as defined in relevant state, commonwealth, or territory nurse practice acts and other applicable laws and regulations, and as permitted by a health care organization in accordance with these definitions.

nursing care Professional processes intended to assist an individual in the performance of those activities contributing to health or its recovery (or to peaceful death) that he or she would perform unaided if he or she had the necessary strength, will, or knowledge. This includes, but is not limited to, assisting individuals in carrying out therapeutic plans and understanding the health needs of individuals. The special content of nursing care varies in different countries and situations, and, as defined, it is not given solely by registered nurses, but also by other health care professionals.

nursing services Services provided to patients by an individual who is qualified by an approved postsecondary program or baccalaureate or higher degree in nursing and who is licensed or certified by the state to practice nursing. These services may be provided directly or through contract with another organization or individual.

nursing staff Registered nurses, licensed practical or vocational nurses, nursing assistants, and other nursing staff who perform nursing care in a health care organization.

nutrients Protein, carbohydrates, lipids, vitamins, electrolytes, minerals, and water.

nutrition The sum of the processes by which one takes in and uses nutrients.

enteral nutrition Nutrition provided via the gastrointestinal tract. Enteral nutrition encompasses both oral (delivered through the mouth) and tube (provided through a tube or catheter that delivers nutrients distal to the mouth) routes.

parenteral nutrition Nutrition provided intravenously to those individuals who have lost gastrointestinal function or who cannot maintain adequate nutrition care status through conventional intake of nutrients. Parenteral nutrition allows safe administration, through a variety of veins, of all daily nutrition requirements to effect protein synthesis and maintain adequate nutrition status.

parenteral product A sterile pharmaceutical preparation introduced into the body through a route other than the digestive tract, as by subcutaneous, intramuscular, or intravenous injection or infusion.

nutrition assessment A comprehensive process for defining an individual's nutrition status using medical, nutrition, and medication intake histories, physical examination, anthropomorphic measurements, and laboratory data.

nutrition care Interventions and counseling to promote appropriate nutrition intake, based on nutrition assessment and information about food, other sources of nutrients, and meal preparation consistent with the individual's cultural background and socioeconomic status. Nutrition therapy, a component of medical treatment, includes enteral and parenteral nutrition. *See also* nutrition.

nutrition screening The process of using characteristics known to be associated with nutrition problems in order to determine if individuals are malnourished or at a high nutrition risk for malnourishment. *See also* nutrition criteria.

occupancy

ambulatory health care occupancy An occupancy used to provide services or treatment to four or more patients at the same time that either

(1) render them incapable of taking their own means for self-preservation in an emergency or (2) provide outpatient surgical treatment requiring general anesthesia.

business occupancy An occupancy used to provide outpatient services or treatment that does not meet the criteria in the ambulatory health care occupancy definition (for example, three or fewer patients at the same time who are rendered incapable of self-preservation in an emergency or are undergoing general anesthesia).

health care occupancy An occupancy used for purposes such as medical or other treatment or care of persons suffering from physical or mental illness, disease, or infirmity; and for the care of infants, convalescents, or infirm aged persons. Health care occupancies provide sleeping facilities for four or more occupants and are occupied by persons who are mostly incapable of self-preservation because of age, physical or mental disability, or because of security measures not under the occupant's control. Health care occupancies include hospitals, nursing homes, and limited care facilities.

residential occupancy An occupancy in which sleeping accommodations are provided for normal residential purposes and include all buildings designed to provide sleeping accommodations.

occupational therapist assistant, qualified, certified An individual who is a graduate of an occupational therapy assistant program accredited by a nationally recognized accreditation body; is currently certified as an occupational therapy assistant by the American Occupational Therapy Certification Board; meets any current legal requirements of licensure or registration or has the documented equivalence in education, training, and experience; and is currently competent in the field. The qualified and certified occupational therapist assistant uses purposeful, goal-oriented activity to assist in assessing, evaluating, or treating persons whose function is impaired by physical illness or injury, emotional disorder, congenital or developmental disability, or the aging process to achieve optimum functioning, to prevent disability, and to maintain health. For purposes of Joint Commission Medicare surveys, occupational therapy assistants meet the personnel requirements as outlined in the Medicare regulations for home health agencies.

occupational therapist, qualified An individual who is a graduate of an occupational therapy program accredited by a nationally recognized accreditation body; is currently certified as an occupational therapist by the American Occupational Therapy Certification Board; meets any current legal requirements of licensure or registration or has the documented equivalence in education, training, and experience; and is currently competent in the field. The qualified occupational therapist uses purposeful, goal-oriented activity in assessing, evaluating, or treating persons whose function is impaired by physical illness or injury, emotional disorder, congenital or developmental disability, or the aging process, to achieve optimum functioning, to prevent disability, and to maintain health. For purposes of Joint Commission Medicare surveys, occupational therapists meet the personnel requirements as outlined in the Medicare regulations for home health agencies.

occupational therapist, qualified, certified An individual who is a graduate of an occupational therapy program accredited by a nationally recognized accrediting body; is currently certified as an occupational therapist by the American Occupational Therapy Certification Board;

meets any current legal requirements of licensure or registration; or has the documented equivalent in education, training, and experience and is currently competent in the field. The qualified occupational therapist uses purposeful, goal-oriented activity in assessing, evaluating, or treating persons whose function is impaired by physical illness or injury, emotional disorder, congenital or developmental disability, or the aging process to achieve optimum functioning, to prevent disability, and to maintain health.

occupational therapy assistant, qualified An individual who is a graduate of an occupational therapy assistant curriculum accredited by a nationally recognized accrediting body or has the documented equivalent in education, training, or experience and meets any applicable requirements for licensure, certification, or registration. For Medicare surveys, occupational therapy assistants meet the personnel requirements as outlined in the Medicare regulations for home health agencies.

occupational therapy services Services that provide for goal-directed, purposeful activity to aid in the development of adaptive skills and performance capacities by individuals of all ages who have physical disabilities and related psychological impairment(s). Such therapy is designed to maximize independence, prevent further disability, and maintain health. These services are provided by a qualified occupational therapist; by a qualified occupational therapy assistant supervised by a registered occupational therapist; or by an individual who has the documented equivalent education, training, or experience and who meets any current legal requirements of licensure or registration. These services may be provided directly or through contract with another organization or individual.

Official Accreditation Decision Report In the Joint Commission accreditation process, the report resulting from the on-site assessment of an organization or network that outlines identified deficiencies in standards compliance. It also outlines the nature of the accreditation decision including enumeration of type I recommendations, the remediation of which will be monitored by the Joint Commission through focused surveys or written progress reports. The report may also include other supplemental recommendations that are designed to assist the organization or network in improving its performance. *See also* accreditation decision; recommendation.

operative and other procedures Includes operative, other invasive, and noninvasive procedures that place the individual at risk. The focus is on procedures and is not meant to include medications that place the individual at risk.

organizationwide Throughout the organization and across multiple structural and staffing components, as appropriate.

orientation A process to provide initial training and information and to assess staff members' competence related to their job responsibilities and the organization's mission, vision, and values.

outcome The result of the performance (or nonperformance) of a function or process(es).

outpatient program A program that provides services to persons who generally do not need the level of care associated with the more structured environment of an inpatient or a residential program.

parenteral nutrition *See* nutrition, parenteral.

parenteral product *See* nutrition, parenteral product.

partial-hospitalization program A program that provides services to persons who spend only part of a 24-hour period in a behavioral health facility. Partial-hospitalization programs do not provide overnight care.

pathology and clinical laboratory services The services that provide information on diagnosis, prevention, or treatment of disease through the examination of the structural and functional changes in tissues and organs of the body that cause or are caused by disease.

patient An individual who receives care or services, or one who may be represented by an appropriately authorized person. Synonyms used by various health care fields include client, resident, customer, individual served, patient and family unit, consumer, or health care consumer. *See also* individual.

performance The way in which an individual, a group, or an organization carries out or accomplishes its important functions and processes.

performance area An element of the Joint Commission accreditation decision grid that summarizes a standard or group of related standards. The performance areas identified on the accreditation decision grid are considered to be the most critical to the final accreditation decision. *See also* accreditation decision grid.

performance improvement The continuous study and adaptation of a health care organization's functions and processes to increase the probability of achieving desired outcomes and to better meet the needs of individuals and other users of services. This is the third segment of a performance measurement, assessment, and improvement system.

performance measure A quantitative tool (for example, rate, ratio, index, percentage) that provides an indication of an organization's performance in relation to a specified process or outcome. *See also* indicator; denominator; numerator.

personnel record The complete employment record of a staff member or an employee, including job application, education and employment history, job description, performance evaluation(s), and, when applicable, evidence of current licensure, certification, or registration.

pharmaceutical care and services Services provided directly or through written contract with another organization that include procuring, preparing, dispensing, and distributing pharmaceutical products and the ongoing monitoring of the individual to identify, prevent, and resolve drug-related problems.

pharmaceutical equivalence The degree to which two formulations of the same medication are identical in strength, concentration, and dosage form.

pharmacist An individual who has a degree in pharmacy and is licensed and registered to prepare, preserve, compound, and dispense drugs and chemicals.

pharmacist, consultant An individual who has a degree in pharmacy and is licensed and registered in accordance with pharmacy law and regulation.

pharmacy A licensed location where drugs are stored and compounded or dispensed.

physical abuse *See* abuse.

physical restraint *See* restraint.

physical therapist assistant, qualified An individual who is educated specifically to work under the direction and supervision of the physical therapist in the delivery of physical therapy services; who is a graduate of a physical therapist assistant associate degree program accredited by the Commission on Accreditation in Physical Therapy Education, a nationally recognized accreditation body, or has the documented equivalence in training, education, and experience; who meets any current legal requirements of licensure or registration;

and who is currently competent in the field. For purposes of Joint Commission Medicare surveys, physical therapy assistants meet the personnel requirements as outlined in the Medicare regulations for home health agencies.

physical therapist, qualified An individual who is a graduate of a physical therapist education program accredited by a nationally recognized accrediting body; who meets any current legal requirements of licensure or registration or who has the documented equivalence in training, education, and experience; and is currently competent in the field. Physical therapists assess, evaluate, and treat movement dysfunction and pain resulting from injury, disease, disability, or other health-related conditions. For purposes of Joint Commission Medicare surveys, physical therapists meet the personnel requirements outlined in the Medicare regulations for home health agencies.

physical therapy aide An individual who is trained on the job to provide support services for the physical therapy department under the direction and supervision of a physical therapist. Direct patient services may include transportation, assistance of other physical therapy staff with dependent patients, and other activities as delegated by the physical therapist. Routine duties of the physical therapy aide include equipment management, preparation and cleaning of treatment areas, and supply inventory.

physical therapy services The health care field concerned primarily with the treatment of disorders with physical agents and methods, such as massage, manipulation, therapeutic exercises, cold, heat (including shortwave, microwave, and ultrasonic diathermy), hydrotherapy, electric stimulation, and light, to assist in rehabilitating individuals and in restoring normal function after an illness or injury.

physician licensure The process by which a legal jurisdiction, such as a state, grants permission to a physician to practice medicine after finding that he or she has met acceptable qualification standards. Licensure also involves ongoing regulation of physicians by the legal jurisdiction, including the authority to revoke or otherwise restrict a physician's license to practice.

physician, qualified A doctor of medicine or doctor of osteopathy who, by virtue of education, training, and demonstrated competence, is granted clinical privileges by the organization to perform specific diagnostic or therapeutic procedure(s) and who is fully licensed to practice medicine.

plan for improvement For purposes of Joint Commission accreditation, an organization's written statement that details the procedures to be taken to correct existing *Life Safety Code®* deficiencies and, where applicable, includes the interim life safety measures to be implemented to temporarily reduce the hazards associated with the deficiencies. *See also* interim life safety measures; *Life Safety Code®*.

plan of correction, conditional accreditation For purposes of Joint Commission accreditation, an organization's written plan, approved by Joint Commission staff, that outlines the actions the organization or network will take to address compliance issues that caused the Joint Commission's Accreditation Committee to make a decision of conditional accreditation. The plan is the basis for the follow-up survey at a specified time once the plan is approved. *See also* accreditation decision.

poetry therapy The initial use of literature or writing by a qualified biblio-poetry therapist to further therapeutic goals and enhance the well-being of individuals through the integration of emotional, cognitive, and social aspects of self.

policies and procedures The formal, approved description of how a governance, management, or clinical care process is defined, organized, and carried out.

preliminary nonaccreditation *See* accreditation decision.

prescribing or ordering Directing the selection, preparation, or administration of medication(s).

primary source The original source of a specific credential that can verify the accuracy of a qualification reported by an individual health care practitioner. Examples include medical school, graduate medical education program, and state medical board.

privileging The process whereby a specific scope and content of client care services (that is, clinical privileges) are authorized for a health care practitioner by a health care organization based on evaluation of the individual's credentials and performance. *See* licensed independent practitioner.

process A goal-directed, interrelated series of actions, events, mechanisms, or steps.

program **1.** An outline of work to be done or a prearranged plan or procedure. **2.** A general term for an organized system of services designed to address the individual's care and treatment needs.

protective services A range of sociolegal, assistive, and remedial services that facilitate the exercise of individual rights and provide certain supportive and surrogate mechanisms. Such mechanisms are designed to help developmentally disabled individuals reach the maximum independence possible, yet protect them from exploitation, neglect, or abuse. Depending on the nature and extent of individual needs, protective services may range from counseling to full guardianship.

provisional accreditation *See* accreditation decision.

psychiatric nurse, qualified A licensed, registered nurse who has a master's degree in psychiatric nursing, who has been certified to practice psychiatric nursing by the voluntary certification process of the American Nurses' Association, or who has the documented equivalent in education, training, or experience.

psychiatrist, qualified A physician who specializes in assessing and treating persons having psychiatric disorders; is certified by the American Board of Psychiatry and Neurology or has the documented equivalent in education, training, or experience; and is fully licensed to practice medicine in the state in which he or she practices.

psychodrama therapy The use of action methods of enactment, sociometry, group dynamics, role theory, and social systems analysis to facilitate constructive change in individuals and groups by developing new perceptions or reorganizing old cognitive patterns and concomitant changes in behavior.

psychologist, qualified An individual who specializes and is licensed in psychological research, testing, or therapy.

Public Information Policy A Joint Commission policy governing the confidentiality or disclosure of information about the performance of a health care organization or network. This policy covers the Joint Commission's performance reports, information publicly disclosed on request, complaint information, aggregate performance data, data released to government agencies, and the Joint Commission's right to clarify information an accredited organization releases about its accreditation status.

qualified individual An individual or staff member who is qualified to participate in one or all of the mechanisms outlined in Joint Commission standards by virtue of the following: education, training, experience, competence, registration, certification, or applicable licensure, law, orregulation.

qualified individual, infection control An individual who is qualified to participate in one or all of the mechanisms outlined in the standards by virtue of one or more of the following: education, training, certification or licensure, or experience. Certification by the Certification Board for Infection Control is often a requirement for infection control practitioners.

quality improvement An approach to the continuous study and improvement of the processes of providing health care services to meet the needs of individuals and others. Synonyms include continuous quality improvement, continuous improvement, organizationwide performance improvement, and total quality management.

quality of care The degree to which health services for individuals and populations increase the likelihood of desired health outcomes and are consistent with current professional knowledge. Dimensions of performance include the following: client perspective issues; safety of the care environment; and accessibility, appropriateness, continuity, effectiveness, efficacy, efficiency, and timeliness of care.

radiologic technologist, qualified An individual who is a graduate of a radiologic technology program accredited by an accreditation body recognized by the U.S. Department of Education; is currently certified as a radiologic technologist by the American Registry of Radiologic Technologists; meets any current legal requirements of licensure or registration; or has the documented equivalent in education, training, and experience; and is currently competent in the field.

reassessment Ongoing data collection that begins on initial assessment, comparing the most recent data with the data collected on the previous assessment.

recommendation A citation requiring corrective action based on the nature, severity, or number of compliance problems which is accompanied by appropriate follow-up monitoring.

type I recommendation A recommendation or group of recommendations that addresses insufficient or unsatisfactory standards compliance in a specific performance area. Resolution of type I recommendations must be achieved within stipulated time frames for an organization to maintain its accreditation.

first-generation type I recommendation The first opportunity an organization surveyed by the Joint Commission has to correct a type I recommendation either through a written progress report or through a focused survey, that is, the first follow-up to a triennial or unannounced/unscheduled survey.

second-generation type I recommendation An organization's second opportunity to correct a deficiency either through a written progress report or through a focused survey, that is, the second follow-up to a triennial or unannounced/unscheduled survey.

third-generation type I recommendation The third opportunity an organization has to correct a deficiency either through a written progress report or through a focused survey, that is, the third follow-up to a triennial or unannounced/unscheduled survey.

supplemental recommendation A recommendation or group of recommendations that encompasses a standard(s) that was scored in less than substantial compliance (that is, less than a score 1) but did not result in a type I recommendation. If not resolved, a supplemental recommendation may affect a future accreditation decision.

recreational therapist assistant or technician, qualified An individual who, at a minimum, is a graduate of an associate degree program in recreational therapy; meets any current legal requirements of licensure, registration, or certification or has the documented equivalence in education, training, and experience; and is competent in the field. Recreational therapy assistants or technicians assist recreational therapists to assess and treat clients individually using interventions to restore, remediate, or rehabilitate to improve functioning and independence in life activities as well as to reduce or eliminate the effects of illness or disability. A qualified recreational therapist clinically supervises the work of recreational therapy assistants or technicians.

recreational therapist, qualified An individual who, at a minimum, is a graduate of a baccalaureate degree program in recreational therapy accredited by a nationally recognized accreditation body; is currently a Certified Therapeutic Recreation Specialist by the National Council for Therapeutic Recreation Certification; meets any current legal requirements of licensure, registration, or certification or has the documented equivalent in education, training, and experience; and is currently competent in the field. Recreational therapists assess and treat clients individually using interventions to restore, remediate, or rehabilitate to improve functioning and independence in life activities as well as to reduce or eliminate the effects of illness or disability.

reference database An organized collection of similar data from many organizations that can be used to compare an organization's performance to that of others.

referral The sending of an individual (1) from one clinician to another clinician or specialist, (2) from one setting or service to another, or (3) by one physician (the referring physician) to another physician(s) or other resource, either for consultation or care.

registered dietitian As defined by the Commission on Dietetic Registration, the credentialing agent of the American Dietetic Association, an individual who completed the minimum of a baccalaureate degree granted by a U.S. regionally accredited college or university; meets current academic requirements (Didactic Program in Dietetics) as approved by the American Dietetic Association; completed preprofessional experience accredited or approved by the American Dietetic Association; successfully completed the Registration Examination for Dietitians; and accrues 78 hours of approved continuing education every five years.

registered nurse An individual who is qualified by an approved postsecondary program or baccalaureate or higher degree in nursing and licensed by the state, commonwealth, or territory to practice professional nursing.

residential occupancy *See* occupancy.

residential program A program that provides services to individuals who need a less structured environment than that of an inpatient program and who are capable of self-preservation in the event of an internal disaster. *See also* inpatient program; outpatient program.

respect and caring The degree to which those providing services do so with sensitivity for the individual's needs, expectations, and individual differences, and the degree to which the individual or a designee is involved in his or her own care decisions.

restraint Any method (chemical or physical) of restricting an individual's freedom of movement, physical activity, or normal access to the body.

chemical restraint The inappropriate use of a sedating psychotropic drug to manage or control behavior.

physical restraint Any method of physically restricting a person's freedom of movement, physical activity, or normal access to his or her body.

risk management activities Clinical and administrative activities that organizations undertake to identify, evaluate, and reduce the risk of injury to clients, staff, and visitors and the risk of loss to the organization itself.

run chart A display of data in which data points are plotted as they occur over time (for example, observed weights over time) to detect trends or other patterns and variation occurring over time. Run charts, as opposed to tabular frequency displays, are capable of time-order analytic studies.

safety The degree to which the risk of an intervention (for example, use of a drug or a procedure) and risk in the care environment are reduced for a clients and other persons, including health care practitioners.

safety management A component of an organization's management of the environment of care program that maintains and improves the general safety of the care environment.

scope of care or services The activities performed by governance, managerial, clinical, or support staff.

second-generation type I recommendation *See* recommendation, second-generation type I.

sentinel event A sentinel event is an unexpected occurence involving death or serious physical or psychological injury, or risk thereof. Serious injury specifically includes loss of limb or function. The phrase "or risk thereof" includes any process variation for which a recurrence would carry a significant chance of a serious adverse outcome.

services Structural divisons of an organization or its staff; also the delivery of care.

significant medication errors and significant adverse drug reactions Unintended, undesirable, and unexpected effects of prescribed medications or of medication errors that require discontinuing a medication or modifying the dose; require initial or prolonged hospitalization; result in disability; require treatment with a prescription medication; result in cognitive deterioration or impairment; are life threatening; result in death; or result in congenital anomalies. *See also* drug; medication.

significant other An individual with whom a patient has a close or formalized relationship, such as a parent, spouse, friend, caretaker, court-ordered fiduciary, or any other person so identified by the parent.

social work assistant An individual with a bachelor's degree, preferably with a social work sequence, who is given training on the job for specific assignments and responsibilities in the provision of social work services or who has the documented equivalent in education, training, or experience. For purposes of Joint Commission Medicare surveys, social work assistants meet the personnel requirements outlined in the Medicare regulations for home health agencies.

social work services Services to assist individuals and their families in addressing social, emotional, and economic stresses associated with illness or injury. Such services are provided by a qualified social worker or a social work assistant under the supervision of a qualified social worker. These services may be provided directly or through contract with another organization or individual.

social worker, qualified An individual who either has met the requirements of a graduate curriculum (leading to a master's degree) in a school of social work that is accredited by the Council on Social Work Education or has the documented equivalent in education, training, or experience. For purposes of Joint Commission Medicare surveys, social workers meet the personnel requirements outlined in the Medicare regulations for home health agencies.

speech-language pathologist, qualified A health care professional who specializes in the measurement and evaluation of language abilities, auditory processes, and speech production; clinical treatment of children and adults with speech, language, and hearing disorders; and research methods in the study of communication processes.

speech-language pathology services Services provided to assist individuals in speech, language, oral and pharyngeal sensorimotor function, cognitive or communicative function, and their underlying processes. Such services are provided by a qualified speech-language pathologist and may be provided directly or through contract with another organization or individual.

speech screening A process to determine language abilities that may include such tests as articulation in connected speech and formal testing situations; voice, in terms of judgments of pitch, intensity, and quality and determinations of appropriate vocal hygiene; and fluency, usually measured in terms of frequency and severity of stuttering or dysfluency (based on evaluation of speech flow-sequence, duration, rhythm, rate, and fluency).

staff Individuals, including employees, volunteers, contractors, or temporary agency personnel, who successfully complete a credentialing process and are granted clinical privileges by the organization.

standard A statement that defines the performance expectations, structures, or processes that must be substantially in place in an organization to enhance the quality of care.

Statement of Conditions™ (SOC™) A proactive document that helps an organization to do a critical self-assessment of its current level of compliance and describes how to resolve any *Life Safety Code*® (*LSC*®) deficiencies. The SOC™ was created to be a "living, ongoing" management tool that should be used in a management process that continually identifies, assesses, and resolves *LSC*® deficiencies.

summary grid score A number that indicates an organization's overall accreditation performance. The grid score is calculated from the grid element scores. Also referred to as the grid score. *See also* accreditation decision grid; grid element score.

supplemental recommendation *See* recommendation, supplemental.

surrogate decision maker Someone appointed to act on behalf of another. Surrogates make decisions only when an individual is without capacity or has given permission to involve others. *See also* advocate; family.

survey team The group of health care professionals who work together to perform a Joint Commission accreditation survey.

surveyor For purposes of Joint Commission accreditation, a physician, nurse, administrator, laboratorian, or any other health care professional who meets the Joint Commission's surveyor selection criteria, evaluates standards compliance, and provides education and consultation regarding standards compliance to surveyed organizations or networks.

tailored survey A Joint Commission survey in which standards from more than one accreditation manual are used in assessing compliance. This type of survey may include using specialist surveyors appropriate to the standards selected for survey.

therapeutic equivalence The degree to which two formulations of different active ingredients are judged by the clinical staff to have acceptably similar therapeutic effects.

therapeutic foster care For purposes of Joint Commission accreditation, intensive services provided to no more than two patients in treatment in a single residence. Services are delivered primarily by treatment foster parents who bear direct responsibility for implementing the select in-home aspects of the treatment plan.

third-generation type I recommendation *See* recommendation, type I.

timeliness The degree to which care is provided to the individual at the most beneficial or necessary time.

transfer The formal shifting of responsibility for the care of an individual (1) from one care unit to another, (2) from one clinical service to another, (3) from one licensed independent practitioner to another, or (4) from one organization to another organization.

treatment plan A plan, based on data gathered during individual assessment, that identifies the care needs of the individual being served, lists the strategy for offering services to meet those needs, documents treatment goals and objectives, outlines the criteria for terminating specified interventions, and documents the individual's progress in meeting specified goals and objectives. The format of the "plan" in some organizations may be guided by individual-specific policies and procedures, protocols, practice guidelines, clinical paths, care maps, or a combination of several methods.

type I recommendation *See* recommendation, type I.

type II recommendation *See* recommendation, supplemental.

utilities management A component of an organization's management of the environment of care program designed to ensure the operational reliability, assess the special risks, and respond to failures of utility systems that support the individual care environment.

utility systems Organization systems for surveillance, prevention, and control of infection; environment support; and equipment support. May include electrical distribution; emergency power; vertical and horizontal transport; heating, ventilating, and air conditioning; plumbing, boiler, and steam; piped gases; vacuum systems; or communication systems including data exchange systems.

utilization management The examination and evaluation of the appropriateness of the utilization of an organization's resources. Also referred to as a utilization review.

variance **1.** A measure of the differences in a set of observations. **2.** In statistics, equal to the square of the standard deviation.

variation The differences in results obtained in measuring the same phenomenon more than once. The sources of variation in a process over time can be grouped into two major classes: common causes and special causes.

waived testing Tests that meet the Clinical Laboratory Improvement Amendments of 1988 (CLIA '88) requirements for waived tests; are cleared by the Food and Drug Administration for home use; employ methodologies that are so simple and accurate as to render the likelihood of erroneous results negligible; or pose no risk of harm to the individual if the test is performed incorrectly. *See also* CLIA '88.

written progress report (WPR) For purposes of Joint Commission accreditation, a postsurvey activity that involves preparing a report documenting evidence that correction of a compliance problem(s) is complete. Preparing a WPR involves summarizing, documenting, and collecting facts and other evidence that prove an organization's current compliance with the standards that caused a type I recommendation. *See also* recommendation.

Index

This index is designed to help the user find items quickly and efficiently. The majority of entries are referenced to specific standards. The standards numbers are listed in parentheses after the page number references. For example, if you are looking for information on assessment of neglect, you would look up "neglect" in this index. Under this heading you would find the subheading "assessment of" and be directed to standards PE.1.18 through PE.1.18.1.3 on page 80.

B

N

O

P

Q

R

T

U

V

W